1 6 OCT

Daisy's GIFT

2 0 DEC 2021
WITHDRAWN
WEST SUSSEX COUNTY COUNCIL

D0239193

Daisy's
GIFT

CLAIRE GUEST

3 5 7 9 10 8 6 4 2

Virgin Books, an imprint of Ebury Publishing,
20 Vauxhall Bridge Road,
London SW1V 2SA

Virgin Books is part of the Penguin Random House group of companies
whose addresses can be found at global.penguinrandomhouse.com

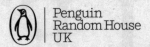

Penguin
Random House
UK

Copyright © Claire Guest 2016

Claire Guest has asserted her right to be identified as the author of this
Work in accordance with the Copyright, Designs and Patents Act 1988

First published in the United Kingdom by Virgin Books in 2016
This edition published in 2017

www.penguin.co.uk

A CIP catalogue record for this book is available from the British Library

ISBN 9780753557426

Printed and bound in Great Britain by Clays Ltd, St Ives PLC

Penguin Random House is committed to a sustainable future for our
business, our readers and our planet. This book is made from Forest
Stewardship Council® certified paper.

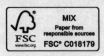

MIX
Paper from
responsible sources
FSC® C018179

This book is dedicated to my mum, my dad, and my sisters Louise, Nicole and Simone, who have supported me all my life. It is also for all the dogs I have loved and who have loved me.

CONTENTS

Introduction

Tail wagging furiously, head cocked and eyes bright, Tangle the chocolate-brown cocker spaniel gazed up at me. 'Let's play!' his face and body language seemed to say.

'Seek, seek,' I said, sweeping my arm away to underline the instruction.

Tangle trotted off and worked his way along a line of stainless steel dishes set out at intervals on the floor. He reached the second from the end and dropped to the ground, head turned to me for approval.

'Good boy,' I said, digging into the bag at my waist for his favourite chewy treat. I bent down to ruffle the soft fur on his head, hoping that my little boy had got it right and had detected, accurately, the presence of bladder cancer in the urine sample he had sniffed. All I knew was that there was one sample from a patient with cancer among the seven, and the other six had been donated by healthy volunteers.

This was a properly conducted scientific trial, and only the scientists and doctors could unlock the codes on the samples to say whether he had got it right. I was confident, but also, naturally, worried.

Tangle and five other dogs were being tested in controlled conditions to assess whether a dog's sense of smell can be harnessed to help humans, not only by sniffing out drugs or explosives, or by guiding the blind along cluttered pavements, or by alerting the deaf to doorbells or telephones, but in a scientific environment, with cancer cells as the target.

There are lots of stories about dogs detecting cancer in their owners. I have one myself: my dog Daisy alerted me to my own breast cancer, which was then successfully treated, but which was so deep that by the time I had found the lump myself it would almost certainly have been too late. But these stories are anecdotal: there was no proper, authenticated proof and, although anyone who was close to a dog was likely to have faith in these accounts, the sceptics could challenge them.

That is why the scientific tests to see if dogs could find cancer in complete strangers were so vital – and, if proved positive, they would help to demonstrate why dogs would, I believe, prove invaluable in the battle to detect cancer early.

The next two weeks were spent on tenterhooks, waiting for the final results of the tests. Then there was the Eureka moment, the phone call that told me our dogs had done it: their success rate was high enough for the prestigious *British Medical Journal* to later accept an article demonstrating the power of dogs' noses in the battle against cancer.

Tangle, who had the best results of the six, spear-headed our breakthrough with the medical profession, and since then we – the scientists, doctors and dog handlers – have been very busy. We have been working long hours to establish that dogs, with noses so many more times sensitive than ours, can become a valuable tool in the detection of different cancers, using entirely non-invasive techniques.

Tangle was a pioneer, the star whose success put a stamp of scientific credibility on our work. His picture went round the world; he appeared on numerous television programmes and gave demonstrations to audiences across the country. His silhouette is immortalised in the logo of Medical Detection Dogs, the charity set up to explore the future of using dogs to alert to cancer.

He took it all in his four-legged stride. He loved fuss and attention but most of all he loved to 'play', and his play was our work.

For me, Tangle's success was something I knew would happen. He was one of my own dogs, an amazing fella who worked his socks off until he retired in 2013, his place now taken by a team of other dogs, all trained to a high level to detect those scents we, as human beings, can-not smell. Sadly, in 2015 he passed on, but he will always be remembered, by me and many others, as the dog who made history.

Everything that has come since that groundbreaking trial, with the setting up of a national charity with the Duchess of Cornwall as our patron, is, for me, the culmination of a lifetime's devotion to animals. More than devotion: an affinity with them that has overridden everything else life has thrown at me.

As a child I endured chronic shyness and at school I was badly bullied; I have had a failed marriage; a massive breakdown that took me to the brink of suicide; breast cancer.

But through everything, I have had dogs. I am now doing my dream job, in charge of the day-to-day running of the charity I helped to set up to train detection dogs. Within a few years, I predict and hope that diagnosis using dogs will be a factor used routinely for a range of cancers.

And as a powerful offshoot, we discovered that dogs can be taught to use their amazing sense of smell to alert people with diabetes when their blood sugars are starting to move from normal, either too high or too low. We are training dogs to live with people with diabetes, and others with diseases like Addison's and nut allergies, giving them peace of mind. Early alerts mean that the number of hospital admissions is hugely reduced, the dangers of collapse are minimised, and the parents of a child with diabetes can sleep at night, not constantly waking every hour or two to monitor their child's blood. The change to their lives, brought by a waggy-tailed, wet-nosed smelling machine, is incredible, and their stories still make me cry, even though I am so aware of what dogs can do.

This is my story: but more than that, it is the story of Ruffles, Dill, Woody, Tangle, Daisy and all the other dogs whose affection and devotion to us, their owners, goes beyond anything we could ever have imagined. Dogs, our loyal, grateful pets, who ask for nothing more than food, a bed and love, will in future be saving even more lives than they already do.

And among the lives they have saved is, without any doubt, mine.

CHAPTER ONE

Ruffles

The advert in the paper said, simply: 'Spaniel needs new home.'

I rang up immediately and went see the dog, and the young family who owned him. He was a beautiful liver and white springer spaniel, about fourteen months old, and completely untrained. They were really struggling with him: they said he was unmanageable, and he was wrecking their house, destroying cupboards, chewing the wallpaper and everything else left within reach. They had two young children and they both went out to work, and they were returning home every day to havoc. He wouldn't walk on a lead, and they were at their wits' end. They were about to take him to the RSPCA rescue centre when I rang up.

I fell in love with him on sight. He was gorgeous, but totally mad. We took him outside the front of their house so that they could show me that he had quite a good recall, and on the way out he knocked over three milk bottles, and tripped the owner up.

I said I would take him, straightaway. He was everything I wanted. His name was Ruffles, which I liked and was very happy to keep.

Ruffles was a very special dog. I have, over the years, owned many dogs, and I've loved them all. But a select few have found their own unique corner of my heart, and will star in my memories for the rest of my life. Ruffles was the first of these wonder dogs.

He was also the dog who reinforced a feeling that was developing strongly in me: I wanted to work with animals.

I was in my second year at university in Swansea when Ruffles came into my life. I had longed for a dog for as long as I could remember but now, having moved out of university halls, I found myself a new place to live. My little flat was in a house in Mumbles, a beautiful, traditional fishing village on the Gower coast, three miles from the university. I was very skinny and fit in those days, as I was often cycling into a head wind along the coast with a backpack full of research material from the library, or running through Singleton Park near the campus.

My landlady was a lovely woman who also had a smallholding a few miles further up the coast at Three Cliffs Bay. I had part of the ground floor of the house, and the great joy was that I had the run of the garden, which backed on to fields.

The landlady was glad to have me, as occasionally I looked after her smallholding at the weekend if she wanted to go away. She was canny: she'd say to me, 'I'm going away this weekend, but I haven't wormed the cats. I'll leave it to you.' Cue me spending the next two days trying to catch the cats, wrap them in towels and get the tablets down their throats. It took hours.

She also had three dogs, so I tentatively broached the subject of having my own dog. She said, 'I'm happy as long as you don't leave him on his own all day while you are at university or all night while you are out.'

Within days, I had Ruffles. From the first day I met him, I was utterly devoted to him, a feeling that was mutual.

Not only was I in love with him, I was also excited at the prospect of trying out my dog-training techniques on him. I was doing a Psychology degree at Swansea primarily because the course included a section on animal behaviour, and this was my main interest. Today, there are universities offering degree courses in animal behaviour studies; in the early eighties this was new territory, but it was territory that fascinated me.

Why? I can't really answer that question. I didn't grow up in a house full of animals, but my parents knew early on that dogs excited me like nothing else: I'd struggle frantically to get out of my pushchair at the sight of a furry, four-legged creature. There was one Dalmatian we passed regularly when I was a toddler, and I'd squeal with joy at the sight of him. Even before I had learned to say many words, I could shout, 'Spotty! Spotty!' Mum and Dad bought me a toy Dalmatian, which, naturally, I called Spotty. It was my favourite toy, and I still have it.

When I was four I decided to leave home, taking my toy Spotty and a bottle of milk I found on the doorstep, and making my way to the house next door. The big attraction was the dog who lived there, a snappy little tan Pembrokeshire corgi who I adored. Looking back, with my dog trainer head on, he was not a child-friendly animal, but to me at the time he was a source of endless fascination. Once, when I bent to stroke him as he lay on his bed, he really snapped at me, enough to put most toddlers off. But I was undeterred.

'I've come to live here,' I told the astonished neighbour who opened the door to my knock. 'I want to live with your dog.'

Kindly, no doubt struggling to suppress a smile, she took me by the hand and led me back home, explaining that I couldn't live with the dog, but that in future if I were good and Mum let me, I could walk him across the fields with her when she went to meet her teenage daughter from school. I was very happy, not just because of the dog, but I can distinctly remember loving being off the pavements and gardens and in wild fields. What could be better than a field and a little dog roaming around at my feet? All my life, I have needed to live near grass and open countryside. After one day in London I am desperate to see a landscape without buildings, topped by a huge, uninterrupted sky.

It wasn't only dogs that held an early fascination for me. At one house where we lived there was an old air raid shelter at the bottom of the garden. Mum and Dad thought I was obsessed with it because I could often be found standing on top of the shelter mound. What they didn't realise, until Dad climbed on the mound himself, was that from my vantage point I could see into a paddock with a pony. I would stand for hours watching the horse, almost in a trance, feeling very calm. I was intensely interested in what he did, which was never more exciting than moving about to fresh grazing. Mum and Dad remember me rushing down the garden whenever I could, and they were amazed at a five-year-old standing still for so long. They were beginning to realise by this time that I had a very special interest in animals.

My desperation for a pet persuaded Mum and Dad to buy me two goldfish, who I named Topsy and Turvy. I was thrilled, loving them as much as it is possible to love two small fish in a bowl. I took my responsibility seriously, cleaning the gravel, changing the water, checking that there was enough weed. But I learned an important lesson from these two hapless creatures: when I went to feed them one morning I found that Topsy had killed Turvy. It's the classic problem of two fish in a small bowl, but I was devastated. I was upset at the loss of Turvy, but also at the realisation that Topsy could do something so terrible. So I learned about the grief that owning pets inevitably brings when they die, but I also realised that you have to understand the world from the animal's point of view: what Topsy did was natural, and was provoked by having to share his territory with another fish. I was only seven, and although I could never have articulated it, I was beginning to understand that animals don't simply behave the way we want them to: they have their own motivations.

Our next family pet was a Pyrenean mountain dog, a beautiful creature we called Angel. Mum and Dad did everything right, researching the breed to be sure they were good around children. They were: they are famously gentle, confident and rarely aggressive with their family, although they make very good guard dogs. They were originally bred to guard the sheep in the mountains, and because they have the same colouring as a sheep they were camouflaged within the flock and able to take any preying wolf by surprise.

We went to the breeder to choose our puppy, and I remember feeling this was the most exciting thing in the world. There was a litter of puppies, and I chose the one who came towards me, with confidence. I knew nothing about dogs or dog training, but it seemed to be a good omen that she was so interested in me.

I remember vividly this white, fluffy bundle arriving, and devoting myself to her. I got up early to spend time with her before school, I groomed her endlessly, I had books about puppies which I read assiduously. I now know that lots of the advice the books gave was wrong: we were told to rub her nose in her mess in order to house train her, which was accepted as common practice at the time. Where did that come from? Which other animal would you train that way?

Dad took her to training classes and, even though I was only nine at the time, I questioned the way there was so much emphasis on dominating her. It was standard dog training in those days, very much in the style of Barbara Woodhouse, the aim being to achieve complete obedience and a master–slave relationship between owner and dog. I couldn't explain it, but it just didn't feel right. Sadly, by the time she was a year old, Angel was having partial seizures, and clearly had a serious problem. Diagnosed with a suspected brain tumour, it would have been cruel to keep her alive because she was suffering. Today, veterinary science could do more for her, but there was no choice back then. We were all very upset, and I remember crying myself to sleep when she had to be put down. I think it put Mum and Dad off having another dog for a few years.

So from very early on in my life , I wanted to be involved in the relationship between dogs and people. I have always found animals easier to understand than human beings. As a child, I lacked confidence around people. Humans were a mystery to me, and I couldn't sense which ones were going to be friendly and which weren't, so they were scary to me. I never had this problem with animals, always being aware what they were thinking and feeling.

It was at university that I discovered by chance that I suffer from a condition known as face blindness (the proper medical name is prosopagnosia), which goes some way to explaining why I find animals easier to read than human beings. Although my face blindness is mild, it means I don't recognise faces, but like most people with the problem, I unwittingly developed lots of strategies to cope. People with face blindness recognise others by their clothes, their gait, their hair colour, their body shape, their voice. I unconsciously use all of these, and on the whole I have always coped very well. But I now know that children with face blindness are often very shy, as I was. I can remember very early in life being very aware of people's shoes. Obviously, individuals change their shoes, but at school less so, and I was probably using this as a clue to their identity.

Having now read a little about it, I was interested to learn that Jane Goodall, the famous primatologist who worked with wild chimpanzees in Africa, is also a sufferer: she, too, has never had a problem recognising animals. I found out about my problem when I volunteered to take part in a study of facial recognition, and failed miserably to recognise and match up any faces.

It seems, looking back, as if so many of my experiences conspired to give me empathy with all animals, but especially dogs. Ruffles gave me the first real chance to try out what I believed, that bullying a dog into submission and becoming the 'top dog' over a dog, which was the fashionable thinking at the time, was the wrong way to go.

Ruffles made it all seem so easy. I was amazed at how quickly he learned everything I taught him. He was a fantastic retriever, he was soon walking to heel, he would stay when I told him. I remember thinking: 'Surely it can't be this easy?'

Looking back, I can see it is odd for a student to have a little spaniel with them at all times, but I never thought about it then.

I had already asked my supervisor if I could bring a dog into uni. The department was very laid back about dogs, because at the time there was an ongoing and groundbreaking study taking dogs into geriatric wards and care homes, to establish whether stroking dogs has a physiological and psychological effect on the heart rates and blood pressure of the elderly people. It sounds so obvious today, but this was the 1980s, and all this work was new – and it was one of the reasons I had applied to go to Swansea.

Roger Mugford, an animal behaviourist who was at the forefront of research into the training of animals, and who is now a good and supportive friend, had in the 1970s carried out with a colleague his 'budgies and begonias' study, in which elderly people living alone were given either budgies or begonias, with a control group being given neither. Following them up proved that the elderly people with the budgies had much greater self-esteem, were happier, had more visitors and used their pet as a conversational gambit to bring them more social contacts than either the begonias group or the controls. These findings had opened the door to the kind of research that was being undertaken at Swansea.

Roger Mugford came to the university to give a lecture to my department, and I was so inspired by him that I went up to talk to him afterwards, and he invited me down to his centre in Surrey. He had just started using a flexi lead – one that extends to allow the dog more freedom but can be retracted again. They were new in this country at the time, and he enthused that they were 'a fantastic bit of kit'. He told me to put a dog on a flexi lead, but I couldn't get the hang of it and the dog quickly wrapped itself around a tree. Roger laughed and said: 'You're a lovely girl, Claire, and I'm sure you'll do well – but not as a dog trainer. I think you should look for another career.'

I've since reminded Roger of this, but he has no memory of saying it. I was mortified at the time, but I was also determined to show him he was wrong. (Years later, he wrote a dedication in the front of one of his books: 'To Claire, the best dog trainer I know.') We giggle about it now.

Before I acquired Ruffles, I made another animal friend. At the start of my second year at Swansea, we psychology students were each given a rat, which we trained using a Skinner box – a chamber inside which the rat learns that by responding to specific stimuli, like a sound or a light, it will get a reward. It can be taught quite complicated sequences. It's how you find out about learning theory.

The rats were issued to us by the university's animal house. We could take our rats home with us if we wanted to, or keep them in the animal house. Mine, which I called Tess after Tess of the d'Urbervilles, one of the Thomas Hardy books that I love, often came home, which some of the other girls who I was sharing with at the time were not too happy about. I had a cage in my bedroom for Tess, and she was very friendly, although you can't have the same relationship with a rat that you can with a dog. I also had a couple of hamsters, which were nothing to do with my university work. They travelled around in my pockets, and I house-trained them. (Recently my life came full circle, when I spent a month socialising a very young hamster that my sister Nicole promised to her nine-year-old daughter Josie for Christmas. I made sure he was used to being handled and wouldn't bite, keeping him in my pocket just like I did at university.)

It was because of one of my hamsters, Asher, that I met another person who influenced my life, and helped propel me towards my future work. When Asher fell ill I was very upset: I'd trained her to do all sorts of things, and I really loved her. I was a typical student, always skint, and I couldn't afford vet fees. But I couldn't see her suffer, so I went to a vet's surgery near to where I was living. It was newly opened, and the vet was a one-man band.

'I'll be absolutely honest: I've got no money,' I said. 'But if you treat my hamster I will come and do anything you want. I'll clean the floor, help out in any way. But please help me.'

Julian Hudson was a great guy, and he did everything he could to save Asher. Unfortunately, because I had unknowingly been keeping her in a cheap Chinese cage, she had stripped the paint off the bars and was suffering from metal poisoning. There was, eventually, nothing more he could do and he had to put her to sleep.

In the meantime, I had started working there, initially just mopping the floor, working out how much dog food was left and doing a bit of filing. But as time went on, Julian trusted me more, and I attended operations, watching to check the animal's breathing while it was under anaesthetic. Julian always talked me through what he was doing. I'd monitor the animals while they were in post-op recovery stage.

Sometimes the work was distressing: I saw dogs suffering from distemper, simply because they had not been vaccinated. But I came to appreciate that it was possible to end an animal's suffering humanely, which we can't do for human beings. It's a terrible decision to have to take, and to this day I dread it, but it is often the right one.

Julian realised I could also help out by sitting with people, particularly elderly ones, after their pets died. He simply did not have time. Often they would tell me their life stories, about their husband or wife dying, their dependence on their pet. On two or three occasions over the time I worked at the surgery I ended up visiting elderly people at home, just to check they were all right. Sometimes they got another pet, sometimes they didn't because they could not face going through another death.

I became even more aware of the very close bond between owners and pets, particularly dogs. I witnessed burly men in tears because their dog was ill. I could see how incredibly powerful these relationships were, and again, looking back, this was a pointer towards my future. I knew then, without being able to articulate it, that we were not using the might of this amazing relationship enough: there was a lot more that dogs could give us, and we could give them.

Julian's wife was a veterinary nurse, and she worked at the surgery whenever she could, and for a time I toyed with the idea of becoming a vet nurse myself. Julian thought this would be a waste, and said that after I had finished my degree I should apply to do a veterinary science degree.

I seriously considered it, because I was already worried about what I would do after university.

Dogs were never far from my thoughts, even though I didn't have Ruffles at this stage. I was aware that nobody was training their rat by bullying it: picking it up and throwing it on the floor, pulling it, standing on its tail. That would not have worked, yet I knew that these were methods people were using with dogs. I couldn't understand: why would we try to dominate and bully an animal that is intelligent, adaptable and programmed to want to please us? Experience showed us that we should teach the rat by reward. I knew from my experience of horses when I was young that you get nowhere by being harsh and bullying them: you have to understand them and work with their personalities.

There was a great deal of talk in the media that dog training was all about control and dominance. They were 'mini wolves', the 'wolf in the living room'. We had long since stopped believing that children should be bullied and beaten, but it was fashionable to think that was how we should treat dogs. Centuries of domestication, of genetically producing an animal that wants to live with us, be with us and do what we want, was thrown over as we went backwards to this nonsense that our pets are wolves.

So that was another reason for me to adopt Ruffles. I knew he was unruly, untrained and his original owners regarded him as 'a problem'. So it was gratifying to be able to train him in a non-threatening way.

Julian looked after all his vet needs, giving him his injections and check-ups, never charging me because I was working without pay at the surgery. Ruffles came into uni with me, I gave him a long run every morning, and in the evenings he came everywhere with me: to the pub, to student parties.

I was at a party one evening and I went to find Ruffles: he was lying on a mattress with a group of young people who were smoking something with a very distinctive aroma. God knows what he inhaled, but he wasn't the worse for it.

He seemed to have an innate sense of what was right and what was wrong. I took him for long walks along the beach, and at that time Swansea beach was plagued by flashers. It was well known: the university authorities warned young female students about it, telling them not to go on the beach alone. It never bothered me, I was happy to ignore these sad individuals. But Ruffles chased them, somehow aware that their behaviour wasn't right.

One of my friends, another psychology student, was interested in studying their behaviour, and wanted to talk to them to try to understand what motivated them. She and I would go down to the beach together, and when we saw a flasher she'd run after him trying to talk, and Ruffles would join her, indignant about his behaviour. I think the combination of the small, cross dog and the mad woman who wanted to analyse them in hot pursuit cleared them from the beach for a while.

Because the university was so close to the sea, we often had beach parties, which Ruffles loved. The other students were happy to lob a ball up the beach for him to fetch endlessly, and he never tired of the game. He only ever switched off at night: the rest of the time he was a bundle of energy.

It was his ability and willingness to retrieve anything that prompted me to look closely at his pedigree, and to read up about what springer spaniels can do. I started entering him for small obedience competitions, and he always won.

The only time we were apart was when I went to lectures: he wasn't allowed to come in with me. But I had a couple of great solutions to this problem. I have, from an early age, loved riding. I was a very shy child: so shy I wouldn't answer the door or pick up the telephone because I couldn't face talking to someone I didn't know. I took it to heart if I was criticised by a teacher or another pupil. I made friends, but I was definitely more interested in animals than people. Riding was a great outlet for me, throughout my childhood.

So at Swansea I was lucky to be put in touch with someone who needed a horse exercising. The stables where the horse lived was a friendly place, and they were happy to let Ruffs stay there for a couple of hours when I was at a lecture.

The other solution was my boyfriend Dave, who had followed me to Swansea and was living in digs working as a landscape gardener, which meant he could sometimes take Ruffles to work with him. I met Dave when I spent a year in Devon, before going to Swansea.

When I was at school, in answer to any question about my future, I always replied that I wanted to work with animals. But I was told rather flatly that the only jobs available were as a kennel maid, cleaning kennels, or a vet, and the A-level requirements for vet school were very high, even above those needed for medical school. I knew, realistically, that I was unlikely to get in, and I had to think hard about what else I could do that would allow me to spend my days with animals. There seemed to be only one other option left open to me: farming.

Eventually, I decided to do a degree course at Seale-Hayne agricultural college in Devon. I was delighted to be leaving Aylesbury, and getting on with my life, and I loved the Devon countryside. If my youngest sister Simone hadn't been in the mix, I would have packed my bags with a light heart, but leaving her was a huge wrench. I was eleven when she was born, and to say I adored her would be an understatement. My other two sisters, Louise and Nicole, were close enough to me in age to be rivals, or simply nuisances. But I fell in love with Simone the minute I saw her. I was never happier than collecting all the bits Mum needed for her: clean nappies, vests, outfits. I helped bathe her, took her for walks, cuddled her; I felt – and I don't mean this in any way disrespectfully, and I know Simone will understand – as though another helpless animal had entered my life, and I would do anything to make her happy.

She was eight years old when I left for Devon. I recently found a heartbreaking letter she wrote to me in her childish handwriting a few months after I'd left, in which she revealed that she'd cried for a fortnight after I went, and carried around with her everywhere four or five books about horses that I had left behind, to remind her of me. I think if anyone had told me at the time that she was crying herself to sleep clutching one of my books, I'd have come straight home.

Before I went, I had to find a placement on a farm near to the college. The practice at Seale-Hayne (which no longer exists as an agricultural college) was for all students to do a year on a farm before studying full time: the idea was to show us a whole run of seasons on a farm, to give a true picture of the life we were choosing. It's a sensible way of making sure you know whether it is the right career. My only experience of farming up to then was potato picking and fruit picking in my school holidays.

It was difficult to find a placement, particularly as a girl, but I was offered one on a mixed arable and dairy farm, which was perfect. I loved being back in the countryside, and before long I was going out with Dave, the farmer's son, a genuinely decent person.

For the first couple of months, the guys working on the farm gave me a hard time: 'Oh my God! It's a girl! Can you drive a tractor? Lift a bale of hay? What are we going to do with a girl?'

However, I was strong and fit, and used to lifting bales of hay for the horses. I'd never driven a tractor, but I was willing to have a go at anything. I took a course of driving lessons in Exeter and, once I passed my test, the farmer insured me to drive all the farm vehicles, including tractors.

This didn't deter the guys on the farm. They laid traps for me: I fell down holes, went down a chute, ended up covered in cow slurry. I got the tractor stuck in slurry and had to crawl out with the muck up to my knees. Every time something happened they said: 'Send us a bloke!' But I think I won them over. On my first trip home, Mum couldn't believe how brown and muscly I was: I couldn't wear feminine tops because I looked like the Jolly Green Giant. I enjoyed the work, picking fruit, collecting eggs. The next-door farm had three hunters which they rode during the winter, and they were pleased to let me exercise them during the summer.

I learned to plough, and I could help with the harvest by rolling, raking and baling. When we did groundwork we drove in a team of four tractors, following each other. The first one was seeding, the next one flattening, the third raking and the fourth hoeing. It was precision work, and by the end the whole field was planted and prepared.

The only problem I had was one that I always have: I am no good at getting up early, and 5.30am milking was a struggle, with me oversleeping a few times. There were between forty and fifty cows to milk, and Dave's dad knew them all by name. He'd tell me to fetch one, and I'd have to cross-check the name with her number, then look for the eartag.

I lived in a lovely room in the farmhouse, and got full board and a little bit of pocket money. I had to go back into college for two or three week-long sessions, filling in work books about what I had been doing, and working on a project.

It was, in many ways, a happy time. But I realised two things in my early farming life. The first was that the animals are cared for well because they represent money, the farm's income. Caring for them is not a matter of respecting and loving them; it is purely financial. If a calf got scour it was a matter of: 'It's not worth getting the vet in.'

The second was that, although I loved helping the cows to give birth, I was very distressed when the calves were taken from their mothers twenty-four hours after they were born. In one part of the farm, the mothers were bellowing and trying to kick the place down, and in another building the calves were crying. I could hear it all from my bedroom window, and it was terrible.

The farmer explained: 'If I leave the calf with the mother, there will be no milk for human beings.'

I understood this, but I wondered why they couldn't be left a bit longer, to have the full benefit of the colostrum that protects them from diseases. Also, at the time I worked there, they were literally pouring milk down the drain to avoid being penalised by the European quota system. I watched it happen, while calves were dying in the shed next door. I understand that it's the way it has to be, but I felt I would never be happy with it.

It was not the relationship I wanted with animals, and I faced a dilemma. If I didn't pursue the agriculture degree, what would I do? Should I take an A level in physics and apply for vet school, or was there something else I should do? By the time I told the college at Seale-Hayne that I would not be coming back, I had already formulated an idea.

On my days off from the farm, I haunted the second-hand bookshops in Exeter, having developed a passion for reading at school. I had a really strong but ill-defined interest in animals: I wanted to work with them, live with them, study them. But I knew I wasn't going to be happy as a farmer or a farmer's wife. At the back of my mind, somewhere deep down, I also knew that being a vet would not satisfy me. But what else could I do?

It was in those bookshops, on the shelves of musty, well-thumbed second-hand tomes, that I first picked up a book by Konrad Lorenz. I had never heard of the famous zoologist and ethologist back then. I didn't even know what an ethologist was: it's a person who studies animals in their natural habitats, rather than in laboratories. Wow! The excitement of reading his early works was like being thumped in the stomach: it took my breath away. I couldn't get enough of his books, and I started to buy anything and everything I could find (or afford) to do with animal behaviour. It felt like coming home: I had known, right from early childhood, that the way to get the best from animals was to understand them, not to impose our wills on theirs, and to encourage from them the behaviour we want. Now I was reading the works of distinguished academics who had spent their lives studying animal behaviour, and their conclusions were the same as mine.

I was really excited about the prospect of getting myself involved in this work, and I began to research how to do it. At that time the main two ways to study animal behaviour at university in the UK were to do a degree in biology or a degree in psychology. Both courses had elements of animal behaviour within them, but I rejected biology straightaway because, having done it at A level, I knew it involved a lot of animal dissection. I wasn't squeamish, but that was not what I was interested in. I wanted to understand the minds of animals, not their physiology.

Human psychology, on the other hand, sounded much more interesting, especially the BSc courses. Some psychology degree courses award a BA, but they tend to be more about social psychology, whereas I was definitely more interested in science-based studies which, in general, included more components of animal learning and training. I narrowed my choices down to two: Nottingham University or Swansea University. Visiting them both, I immediately knew I wanted to go to Swansea. It's by the sea, the surrounding countryside is staggeringly beautiful and the university is not in an enclosed city-centre environment.

The problem was that by the time I realised what I wanted to do, I had missed the UCCA application window (the Universities Central Council on Admissions, which back then was the body that allocated students to courses across the UK). I was really despondent about this as I didn't want to take a year out, having already spent a year in Devon. Mum came to my rescue. She spoke to a friend of hers, the headmaster of the boys' grammar school in Aylesbury, who told me to write a letter to the head of the psychology department at Swansea, and said that he would make a phone call on my behalf. I was astonished. 'You mean I don't have to go through UCCA?'

'They can make their own decisions, you know,' he said.

It worked, and I was invited down for an interview. I was very nervous, but when I look back I can see that when the head of department asked me why I wanted to study psychology, and followed up with why did I want to come to Swansea, I was equipped to answer both questions perhaps better than many of the eighteen-year-olds who had just finished their A levels. I was very enthusiastic, and I think it showed.

So that's how I came to Swansea, and how I met Ruffles.

When I first got him, I thought I would use him in the ongoing study into the effects dogs have on human heart rates and blood pressure, and conversely the effects of stroking and being affectionate with a dog on the dog's heart rate and blood pressure. He did help out with the study: his tail never stopped wagging when the elderly people made a fuss of him, all of them wearing monitors that showed their blood pressure and heart rate dropping. But in my third and final year, when I had originally expected I would join this research, I decided instead to look at aggression in animals, a subject that fascinated me. I was interested in whether adding soya to dog food makes dogs more or less aggressive. Mice, like dogs, are social animals, and they defend their own territory in much the same way that dogs do, so they were the obvious choice for the study. Soya provides phytoestrogens, plant-based hormones. My instinct was that, as oestrogens are female hormones, the addition of soya should make dogs less aggressive. But my research lecturer told me that subtle amounts of oestrogen break down in male bodies as testosterone, and can actually make animals more aggressive.

I studied my mice closely, using a video to record their behaviour when in contact with a new mouse. At the end of the study I demonstrated that the mice fed with soya were more aggressive than those on a different diet. Of course, my research did not lead to any application: I think there has recently, almost thirty years later, been a research project looking at the same thing. There is still a soya component in most dog foods.

When the project was over, to my horror I discovered that my mice, the ones I had been studying, would all be gassed in the animal house because they could not be used for other research. I could not bear the idea of sending them to the gas chamber, so I took them home with me – all fifty of them. They were sweet little white mice, with pink noses and pink feet. I was harassing everyone I knew: 'Would you like a mouse? They're very well behaved ...'

I managed to find homes for most of them, and kept a few myself, probably increasing the popular perception that I was a mad animal person.

After graduation, Ruffles and I moved back home to the family home in Aylesbury; but I was looking for the next opportunity.

CHAPTER TWO

Working with Dogs at Last

I t was a warm homecoming. Simone was thrilled that I was back, and also thrilled with Ruffles, who had been there before during my holidays, but now moved in. The family Labrador, Liza, and Ruffles got along fine, and, although living in Aylesbury was too urban for me, it was lovely to be back with my family. We are and have always been a very close unit, with a shared sense of humour, shared jokes, and a very strong commitment to looking out for each other.

But that didn't mean I could freeload.

'You can't sit around here for months,' Dad said, so I set about looking for a job.

I found one at the timber preservation department of the Building Research Establishment, which in those days was a government organisation doing research, consultancy and testing for the construction industry (it still exists, but is now a charitable trust). The BRE had a laboratory at Princes Risborough, not far from where I was living, where research was being carried

out into ways to improve the tensile strength and dura-
bility of different timbers. It was interesting work: we
would treat samples of wood in the lab with different
chemicals, then take them out into the local woods and
forests and leave them in places of varying dampness
and temperatures, going back at intervals to monitor
the rot and damage, to assess which treatments were the
most effective.

My boss was a lovely guy, good to work for. The work
suited me, as I had always enjoyed chemistry, and this
involved understanding the chemistry of how additives
were increasing the strength of the wood and stopping rot.
I learned how to pressure treat wood. Most of all I loved
the fact that I could get out of the lab into the countryside, taking Ruffles with me.

My boyfriend Dave moved back to Buckinghamshire
with me, and soon after my return we moved in together.
He was again working as a landscape gardener, and in
some ways I was happy. Dave is a good man, a kind and
considerate companion. We bought a little two-bedroom
starter home in the pretty village of Steeple Claydon;
I was doing a job I enjoyed; I could work flexitime so
that I could always fit in a good run with Ruffles; and I
remember Dad extolling the virtues of working in what
was effectively a civil service post, with its security and
index-linked pension, and a good structure of career
progression. I was out in the countryside again, and
although it was not as beautiful as my beloved Dorset,
where we lived until I was a teenager, the Chilterns were

growing on me. Added to all this was the bonus of being back near my family. Mum and Dad were always happy to look after Ruffles for me if I was going to be tied up in the lab all day.

I drove a little Fiat 126, known to my friends as 'the roller skate', and I could wind the roof right back in good weather, knowing that Ruffles would never think of jumping out.

Was this enough for me? Was it a good idea to give up a job I enjoyed to go back to Swansea to become a student again, doing a masters degree in animal behaviour, which was an option I was considering? Maybe, I told myself, I can settle for this, knowing that I was lucky to have a job I liked, a partner who was supportive, and a dog I deeply loved.

Maybe. But one lunchtime from work I took Ruffles for a walk up into the Chiltern Hills near Bledlow Ridge. It was a dull day, but the views were still spectacular. I paused to take them in, and as I stood there, with Ruffles snuffling at the undergrowth, the clouds parted and the sun streamed through. Suddenly I was flooded with a very strong emotion, the intensity great enough to have seared it into my memory. I knew, with deep conviction, that my life was going to change, and that it needed to change. Training Ruffles and looking after him was very satisfying, but it was definitely not enough. I had to work with animals; it was what my life to this point had been about. I could not trade my hopes and ambitions for a pension and a cosy life.

There was something about the feeling that told me that the coming change was a certainty: I was heading towards it and it was out of my hands. At first I assumed it meant I should definitely go back to university. But three days later I realised that it was something else: I saw an advert in the local paper for an assistant dog trainer to work at a new charity, Hearing Dogs for the Deaf. The charity was in its infancy, having been founded two years earlier to replicate work done in the USA. It had only recently begun placing dogs to live with people who had hearing impairment. The dogs were trained to alert their owners to the telephone, the doorbell, the smoke alarm and other normal noises around the house or in the local environment.

The job paid half the money I was getting, it had no pension, there was no flexitime, no stability, and I would get only one weekend off in four. The other three weekends I had to run the kennels where the dogs lived. On lots of levels it didn't make sense, but to me it was a natural fit. We could just about manage to pay the mortgage with my reduced money, and Dave was, as ever, supportive, saying: 'It's what you've always talked about.'

To me it was very appealing. I would be working with dogs. I would also be able to use my experience training rats and mice: I had taught rats to respond to sound stimuli, and I knew if I could do it with a rat I could certainly do it with a dog. What's more, the work was helping people, and I always believed that the strong bond between dog and man had not been tapped.

The chief executive of the fledgling charity was Tony Blunt, an ex-police dog trainer. He was a fantastic boss, and happily took me on straightaway as his assistant trainer. I was only the fourth member of staff to join. When we first met, Tony said to me, 'I love your expertise. We are really going to make a difference.'

Taking the job at Hearing Dogs was a massive milestone for me, one of the truly wonderful breaks I have had in my life. I was evangelical about the work we did. I loved every minute of it. Ruffles came to work with me, and I very quickly trained him as a demonstration dog. Being such a new organisation, it was important to keep raising funds, and at evenings and weekends I'd toddle off to give talks to Women's Institutes, scout groups, anyone who would listen. Although I was still basically shy, I have always been able to overcome it when I am enthused by the subject I'm talking about: I concentrate on what I'm saying, not the audience. It's as though my passion for the subject takes over. Although I find it very difficult to walk into a party on my own, or meet someone in a pub full of strangers, standing up to address a big audience about dogs is completely different. Ruffles would also come along and show them how he could respond to a whole variety of sounds, and he always stole the show.

I loved taking the dogs to their new homes, and watching them settle in, instantly making life-changing improvements to the lives of their new owners. I never grew tired of seeing the bond between them develop: to this day I'm moved beyond words when I see a dog looking after an owner, whether it's a guide dog, a hearing dog, a dog helping a person with disabilities or – and this is the really special bit – doing the job we now train them for, saving the lives of people with diabetes and other people with life-threatening diseases. But that's the future.

I was able, at Hearing Dogs, to put my theories about dog training into practice, and as Tony became more absorbed with the administration of a rapidly growing charity, he was happy to let me get on with it.

We had sixteen weeks to train a dog to recognise six sounds, and at first this was tough, as the dogs came from rescue centres. Later the charity started its own puppy-walking scheme, and these dogs were easier to train as we had input with them while they were socialised. I developed my own methods of evaluating the behaviour of dogs in rescue centres, based on assessments that are used in human psychology. Although there are thousands of nuances in human personality, they can be factored down to a small number of core traits, and I realised that the same applies to dogs.

There's a problem with using the words 'neurotic' and 'psychotic' for both dogs and humans, because we tend to use them as pejorative terms and associate them with mental illness. But they are in fact a continuum, and the mental illness only comes at the extreme edges. Most behaviours can be factor analysed into two groups, each of two behaviours: psychotic/neurotic and introvert/extrovert. There is a whole band of 'normal neurotic' and 'normal psychotic' behaviour, with the neurotics being worriers, carers, interacting with those around them, learning quickly from their experiences. The psychotics are more daring, take chances, don't need to function as part of a group. They are thicker-skinned, and don't learn so well from experience. In terms of training dogs, it is easier to work with those with neurotic traits, and this tends to go with certain breeds. Fighting dogs, for example, are more likely to have psychotic traits, whereas spaniels and Labradors, the breeds most often used for training, are generally on the neurotic spectrum.

As far as the introvert/extrovert division goes, introverts tend to be uncomfortable with social bonding, don't join groups and become isolated. Extroverts gain confidence from those around them, they are curious and look about them, and they want to be part of a group.

So the best combination for training is a dog with neurotic/extrovert tendencies, but never too far along either axis, and that's what I look for.

When I meet a dog I can quickly assess it. The first thing to note is how it interacts with me: I'm looking for a dog that is interested, but not clinging. I want it to look me in the eye. There is an old theory that if a dog looks you in the eye it is trying to dominate you, but that's just not true. It is looking to see what you want. Dogs read our emotions, they are checking in with us all the time. A good dog to train is one that takes an interest in me, but then moves off to look round the room because he's interested in other things, but comes back to me to check in.

If they are puppies, or small breeds, I pick them up and feel their body tension. Are they uptight? Are their neurotransmitters firing rapidly? At first, if you lift a pup away from its mother, its heart rate will go up. But I'm interested in its recovery rate, how quickly it then relaxes, with the heart rate going down, or if it stays in a heightened state of anxiety. We need calm dogs to train, not fearful dogs that are too far along the neurotic spectrum. If the dog is too big to pick up, I hold it and I can, again, assess its tension.

Working at Hearing Dogs felt like coming home to me, and I was happy to abandon my plans of going back to Swansea to do a masters degree: I later did my masters as an external student at Warwick University, carrying out a longitudinal study into the psychological effects that a hearing dog has on its new owners. Not surprisingly, my conclusion was that owners became happier, more sociable, less anxious, less depressed and more energetic, and this change in their mood was still there eighteen months after the dog's arrival in their life, which was the length of time I studied. (My study took almost seven years, and was not published until 2006.)

Not only had I found a job I loved, but I also met a great friend, whose influence on my life has been profound. Gill Lacey was the placement counsellor at Hearing Dogs, and had been there from the charity's beginning, placing the first dogs in the community with people with hearing loss. She shares my devotion to dogs, and we often spent our lunchtimes together chatting over our sandwiches. Very soon after we met, Gill told me a story about herself that struck a deep chord with me, and which is one of the foundation blocks on which all the important work we do now is based. We discussed it endlessly.

When she was in her late teens and living at home, she was very close to the family's pet dog, a Dalmatian bitch called Trudie. The dog started licking a very small mole on Gill's leg, becoming obsessive about it to the point of really annoying her.

'Get off, leave me alone,' she would say, pushing her off. But Trudie came back. And back. And back, so that even when she was asleep in her basket Gill would try to tiptoe past, but she would always wake, put her nose in the air, and then pursue Gill to start licking again. Eventually Gill went to her doctor, who removed the mole, telling her that it would be sent away for tests, but was very unlikely to be anything sinister because skin cancer is very rare in teenagers and young adults (fewer than 1 per cent of all cases). The dog immediately forgot about her leg. It was ten days later that the phone call came: the lab results on the mole showed it was a malignant melanoma. Luckily, it had been completely removed, and Gill's life was safe. Trudie had saved her: the melanoma would have invaded her body by the time she found it without the persistent licking.

She and I both believed that the dog was able to smell the disease, that it recognised this mole was different to any other by its odour. We talked endlessly about how this super-smell ability could be harnessed, but we weren't able, then, to do more than speculate. What if Gill's family hadn't owned a dog? What about all the cases that are not diagnosed until too late, which a dog would have been able to find? It seemed to us both that we were wasting the valuable skills that dogs could bring to human lives. As we knew from Hearing Dogs, the animals we have bred for centuries to be our best friends have an enormous amount they can give us in return for our love and care.

I have a great deal to be grateful to Gill for. I had very bad toothache one day, and I knew it was because of my wisdom teeth. When I was at university I had twice failed to turn up for operations to remove them, simply because I was terrified of anything that involved needles and medical treatment. Gill's partner Mike is a dentist, and she explained to me that he worked with someone who specialised in nervous patients, and that they may be able to do it in the dentist's chair, rather than me being anaesthetised in hospital.

I tried to prepare myself by reading up in my psychology books about desensitisation, but I was still a gibbering wreck when the day came. I was put on a Valium drip, and eventually all four teeth were removed. But Mike told me afterwards that he had never seen anyone as nervous as me, and that they had almost had to abandon the job. I don't remember, but he told me I was pushing him away, and pushing his equipment out of my mouth.

'You really need some help,' he said.

I decided against therapy, but with Mike's help I desensitised myself, using the same techniques I'd use with a dog. For several days before a trip to the dentist I'd practise relaxation, and, having now had a positive experience, I'd build on that to prepare me. On every visit I took less and less Valium, until I no longer need it for a routine check-up.

It was in my early days at Hearing Dogs that I acquired Minstrel. I wanted the challenge of training a breed that had a reputation for being difficult to train, and I knew that flat-coated retrievers were renowned for being more tricky, but still trainable. I bought Minstrel, a liver-coloured puppy, from a GP who loved flat coats and had bred a litter from a working dog line. When I went to look at the litter I couldn't choose between the puppies: by contrast, I've had experiences later, with Dill and Woody and Daisy, when I've known straightaway which puppy I wanted. But when I was doing the paperwork to buy Minstrel he managed to get his tail caught in the door, which gave him a permanent little nobble on his tail, but he hardly complained. Something about his clumsiness and his cheerfulness cemented the bond between us. He was, indeed, a lot more resistant to training than Ruffles, and was quite a wilful dog, so I learned a great deal about perseverance from him.

He came into my life as a nine-week-old puppy, but it was a very difficult time for me, because shortly afterwards Ruffles had an incident that was to have far-reaching consequences.

One day I was taking him for a walk at lunchtime and I didn't realise there was a dog, a collie, tied up in the boot of a car, which had the boot lid up. As we walked past he leaped, snarling, at us, slipped his collar and descended on Ruffles in a fury, tearing his face to shreds. I have never seen such a frenzied attack in all my years of working with dogs. I could see chunks of flesh being torn off and flung to the floor. The owner was screaming, kicking and hitting her dog. By the time she got him off, one side of Ruffles's face was hanging off.

I rushed him to the vet's and he went straight into the operating theatre. His face was sewed back together, although he had a large scar for the rest of his life and the fur down it grew back white. There was a danger that he would lose one eye, but the vet was able to save it, thankfully.

Ruffles was pumped full of antibiotics. I was distraught: he had been my companion for so long. Then while he was still on antibiotics we found an abscess on the back of his neck, caused by dirt getting into his wound during the fight, so he had to go back into the operating theatre. The other dog's owner blamed me completely for walking past her car with a male dog when I knew that hers was aggressive …

Today my friends and family think I have an aversion to all collies. I realise that you can't condemn the whole breed because of one dog, but I do tend to avoid them when I'm out walking my dogs. In one very small way I am grateful to the dog that attacked Ruffles: he made me look at the issue of poor impulse control in dogs, which leads to aggression and is behind almost all serious problems with dogs.

Impulse control should be taught from early in a puppy's life. It's a skill its own mother would teach it: if the bitch has whelped in good conditions, with a stable temperature and plentiful food, she will, after a few weeks, start telling her puppies off when they try to suckle and she doesn't want them to, or if they annoy her in some way. Today we take puppies from their mothers quite early, which is good for socialising them, but they may not have had time to learn this impulse control from their mothers. There's a risk that the human owners will not teach them control because the puppies are cute and small, and are allowed to get away with anything. At this stage it is vital they learn to understand 'no'. Trying to stop a behaviour they've been allowed to do as pups, but which is unacceptable when they are bigger, is much harder than nipping it in the bud when they are very young. If the owner doesn't teach them this, then the dog has never learned to think: 'I'd like to do that, but I can't.'

It is easy to teach a puppy that no amount of scratching the hand or barking will release the treat that is in the hand. The treat will only be given when he sits quietly and calmly. Then he will realise he is being rewarded for the change in his emotional state, which is basic impulse control. The owner has to start this training early, giving the dogs the basic building blocks of control, so that later, when he faces much greater temptations than a treat, he will respond to being told no.

While he was still recovering, and soon after I got Minstrel, I waited for my usual early morning wake-up call: Ruffles jumping on to the bed. He didn't come. This was very unusual, and when I got downstairs I found him vomiting and lying in a pool of bloody diarrhoea.

I knew this was very serious, not just a tummy upset, so I rushed him to the vet where he was diagnosed with parvovirus. Parvo is a viral infection first found in the UK in the late seventies, but it was not until much later in the eighties that vaccination against this deadly killer became widely available. Both Ruffles and Minstrel, the tiny puppy, had been given the vaccination, but the heavy doses of antibiotics Ruffles was on as he recovered from the attack had probably prevented it taking. He was very ill.

After the third day, I was at work when I took a truly terrible call from the vet's surgery. Ruffles was too far gone to save, there was nothing more they could do. They would wait until I went in to say goodbye, then they would put him down.

Gill, my great friend and colleague, adored Ruffles, and she was very upset by the news.

'Have they tried everything?' she said. 'It's worth ringing Bruce Fogle.'

Bruce is a well-known vet, the author of many books about dogs, and a trustee and co-founder of Hearing Dogs. I was reluctant to ring him because, although I did not know the vet practice where Ruffles was being treated very well, I felt I had to defer to their medical expertise.

Gill persisted. 'Don't give up on Ruffles. Ring now, come on.'

So I did. I told Bruce that Ruffles had definitely tested positive for parvo, but when he asked me what treatment he had been given I couldn't answer about specific drugs. I rang the vet and asked for the information. They were very reluctant to give me the details, but in the end I found out that Ruffles had not had all the drugs Bruce would have put him on. When I rang Bruce back, he said: 'You've got to move him. I'm not promising he can be saved, but he hasn't had everything he could have. I have a very good friend in Aylesbury, a vet who will do everything for him. If Colin Price can't save him, nobody can.'

I rang the vet where Ruffles was being treated, and they told me I could not take him home: he was too ill to move, I was being irresponsible. If I took him away he would die, and they had an obligation to put him to sleep on site, humanely.

I spoke to Bruce again who told me to turn up and take my dog. It wasn't easy. Poor old Mum sat in the car outside, with the engine running, like a getaway driver in a gangster movie. I went in and asked for Ruffles.

'You can't take him,' said the receptionist.

'I can, he's mine.'

The altercation went on for a minute or two, then I simply barged through the door to the kennels at the back. Ruffs saw me and, bless him, stood up and wagged his tail, then slumped down, unconscious. I opened the cage and lifted him out, complete with his drip: Bruce had told me not to remove it.

I wrapped him up, well aware how contagious parvo is, and Mum drove as fast as she dared to the new vet. I genuinely thought he may have died as I held him, he was so still and his heartbeat imperceptible. As soon as we arrived, Colin Price was ready, feeling for his pulse and giving instructions to his team for fluids, adrenalin and other drugs.

As he took Ruffs from me, he looked at me and said: 'I will do my best. He's pretty far gone, but we're going to give him a chance.'

He told me to burn the blanket and my clothes, and to disinfect the car. I hardly slept, crying all night and blaming myself for inadvertently causing him suffering. When the phone rang the next morning I had prepared myself for the worst.

'He's taken two litres of fluid, he's still with us, he's a strong dog,' Colin said. He explained that the most important thing was to keep high levels of fluid going in and wait for the virus to pass.

He was in hospital for two weeks, and when he came out he was still not parvo clear. I wasn't able to bring him home at first, because I was working with dogs and there was a danger of cross-contamination, but a wonderful friend looked after him until the great day when he was allowed back to me.

Colin Price is a hero to me. He has now retired, but his practice is run to the standards he set. We still take our dogs there, and they refer very quickly to specialists if there is a problem they can't deal with.

Ruffles bounced back, and continued to work as a demonstration dog for Hearing Dogs for the rest of his life. But there was one side effect: his digestive system was compromised, and from that point on he could only eat fish and rice, supplemented by multivitamin tablets. Every time we tried to introduce something new into his diet, he had terrible diarrhoea. So everywhere I went I had containers full of smelly fish and rice, and I'm sure when I met people they could smell it on me. I did more cooking for Ruffles than I did for us.

Minstrel the puppy was tested for parvo as soon as Ruffles was diagnosed, and Colin continued to test him at intervals, but he remained clear. I was warned that if he vomited or had diarrhoea, I had to take him in immediately, as these were the first signs. So when he was sixteen weeks old and I found him doing squittery, messy poos everywhere, it was straight into the car and down to the vet's.

'He's not well – but he did eat a handkerchief yesterday,' I said to Colin.

Colin looked at me resignedly – but at least the large handkerchief the tiny puppy had swallowed was better than the parvovirus. It was a harbinger of things to come: I soon discovered that Minstrel loved eating anything that had my odour on it. Socks and knickers were his favourites. It was an irritating and dangerous habit, though it was always hard to be cross with such a loveable clown as Minstrel.

On one occasion I was very ill with flu, feeling really rotten, when I realised Minstrel had knocked the top off the linen basket and had a feast on my clothes. He was bored: I was too ill to take him for a good walk.

I rang the vet: 'I'm really ill with flu. I'm pretty sure my flat coat has eaten some clothing.'

'What's he eaten?'

'I think it's a couple of pairs of socks and some knickers …'

'Bloody hell, bring him in. That's too much.'

He was given emetic injections and we all watched while, to my shame, he brought up three pairs of knickers, including my favourite pair. Everyone was crying with laughter. They knew me as a dog trainer from Hearing Dogs, and by this time I had made a bit of a name for myself as a canine behaviourist: and here I was, with a dog eating a large part of my underwear collection.

He did it all his life, and it got to the point where, if it was only one sock or one pair of knickers, I didn't take him to the vet but simply waited for nature to take its course.

He was, as I anticipated, a very difficult dog to train. I had to repeat everything to him endlessly, and began to fear that he would never get it. He'd give me a strange quizzical look, as much as to say: 'Am I supposed to be following this?' Then he'd look away again, and I'd be begging him to listen to me.

On one occasion he nearly drowned when he was supposed to be taking part in a gun-dog trial. Ruffles was competing at the top of his game, and everyone admired him, but Minstrel would either perform really well, or else he seemed determined to make an idiot out of me. On this particular occasion, a woman who was interested in flat coats asked if she could come and watch him compete. He was supposed to look at me to watch what he was supposed to do, but he was water mad and he plunged into a lake, with no idea where the dummy that he was supposed to retrieve had gone. He was so excited to be in the water that he was splashing about chaotically, not responding to my whistles or commands. Eventually he must have realised, in that woolly brain of his, that I was blowing the whistle and he turned to look at me with that 'What, me?' expression on his face.

He was a very amiable dog, not frightened of anything. I think you could have exploded a bomb near him and he would have been unperturbed. Most dogs have an instinctive fear of the unknown, but Minstrel went straight for it. He was attracted to unusual-looking people: when we were out walking he'd head straight for anyone that common sense told me we should be giving a wide berth.

He loved jumping up at people, and being a large dog he gave one or two people a nosebleed with his exuberance. I did eventually get him trained to a reasonably high level, but it was hard work. Whenever I'm called in to help with the training of a badly behaved pet, I try not to be critical of the owners: I know just how difficult it is with some dogs. I simply encourage them to persevere and give the right amount of time to the training.

Ruffles and Minstrel got on very well. They were like Morecambe and Wise, a real double act. Ruffs was the brains: I could see him looking at me for my response when Minstrel did something naughty.

'Uh, uh, Minstrel's in trouble again …' his face said.

There was nothing malicious or unpleasant in either of their characters, but Minbag (as my dad called him) could be relied upon to wreak havoc, knocking into things and flattening all around him. His enthusiasm for life never dimmed.

Some time later, when we were living in a small village, there was a spate of break-ins one night. Ours was the last house at the end of the village, and we were woken up by Ruffles, nudging me, trying to tell me something, clearly very upset. He started barking, and kept rushing backwards and forwards from the bedroom window to the bed, so I staggered into wakefulness and went to look. Below, on the road, I could see two figures trying to break into my car. I shouted at them, then rushed downstairs and opened the door for Ruffles and Minstrel to go out.

'Go get him, Ruffs!' I shouted. He shot out and grabbed the trouser leg of one of the thieves, who struggled to shake him off. Ruffles meant business. At that moment, Minstrel, the big, blundering retriever, came dashing out, thrilled, convinced this was some new game. He was delighted to meet a couple of unannounced strangers in the middle of the night, and in his enthusiasm to greet them he managed to trip one of the men up as they tried to run away, then kept knocking into them. They were clearly terrified of him, unaware that as far as he was concerned they were great fun and it was all incredibly exciting. Ruffles, the small spaniel, was the one they should have been scared of, but Minstrel's size and clumsiness were too much for them.

The police had been called before the men got as far as our house, by others further up the village, and I could hear the sound of their cars approaching. It was pitch black, and the thieves managed to run off, with the dogs in hot pursuit, plunging into a ditch to hide. I called Ruffles and Minstrel back, afraid they would be hit by a police car. The men did not move, clearly terrified that the dogs were going to find them. I heard one of them say: 'The dogs are still out!'

So it wasn't too difficult for the policemen to make the arrests, and Ruffles and Minstrel were the heroes of the hour. Minstrel was so excited that he jumped up and nearly took a policeman's eye out.

Ruffles and Minstrel both lived until they were fourteen and a half years old, Ruffles dying five years before Minstrel.

Ruffles was a real old man by the time he died. His heart was still good, but he was having trouble walking and he was losing control of his bladder and bowels. A nice young vet came to our house and put him to sleep in the living room, with me holding him. Because of his stomach problems, he was never allowed to have chews, which he coveted when he saw other dogs having them. So I gave him a great big chew, and he died with it in his mouth, very happy.

We buried him under the cherry tree in the garden, but I grieved so badly for him that at night I would howl with anguish, and all I wanted to do was dig up his body so that I could hold him again. The feeling was so powerful it completely flattened me: I hadn't expected to feel so strongly. When we take on dogs, we know they will probably die before we do; it's part of the deal. But it has never been easy.

Ruffles was my first dog, a very special dog, the one to whom, probably above all others, I owe my life's work.

The bond we had was so great that my mourning for him was visceral, I felt as if part of my body had been torn away.

When Minstrel died, I had him cremated and buried his ashes with his dear friend Ruffles, under the cherry tree.

CHAPTER THREE

A House Full of Dogs

About a year after I joined Hearing Dogs, my personal life changed. By then I had been promoted to trainer, and we took on another assistant dog trainer, Andy. His attitude to dogs and their training dovetailed with mine, and it soon became apparent to both of us that we were going to be more than just colleagues. I told Dave straightaway: splitting from him was sad but inevitable, and I knew it was important to be honest. Our relationship was companionable, but never exciting: we were like an old married couple, not two young people in our twenties. The break-up was as amicable as possible, and I am still friendly with Dave, but I was very upset for him at the time and there was a lot of angst and guilt involved. He accepted the inevitable, and it's a tribute to him that he said: 'You won't be happy if you stay here, and I can't keep you here. I'll be all right.'

Andy and I worked side by side every day: it takes two people to train a hearing dog, one to hold the dog and one to set off a sound, putting it very simply. We spent almost every weekend on duty at the Hearing Dogs kennels, covering both our shifts there, because if we worked together we finished more quickly and had time for long country rambles with my dogs. We rented a house for a year, while we discussed our future, moving in with Ruffles and Minstrel. I was twenty-eight, but I felt a failure in some ways because of hurting Dave.

The feeling of guilt was counter-balanced by the belief that I had met another soul mate, but this time a human being not an animal, and my relationship with Andy was blissfully, intensely happy. We talked for hours about dogs and dog training, and we were both agreed that there was some very bad, domineering dog training going on in Britain at the time. We were evangelical: we were going to help change the world and make it a happier place for dogs.

We married, in 1991 when I was thirty-one, after being together three years. We bought a house in a village in Oxfordshire, but soon saw an advert for a canalside cottage, near Tring in Hertfordshire, which was being sold by British Waterways. We had to drive down the towpath to get to it, and as soon as we saw it I fell in love with it. I walked into the kitchen, looked at the view from the window, and knew we had to have it. For the first time since I left Dorset as a teenager, I no longer felt I wanted to go back there. This cottage, and our life together, was perfect.

Buying it was very straightforward, and we got it at a reduced price because it needed a lot of work doing. We had to have it treated for woodworm and damp-proofed professionally, but we worked on the rest ourselves, spending all our free time painting. I replaced or repaired all the woodwork on the window frames myself: I knew I should have done woodwork at school. (I wanted to, but the school insisted it was a boys' subject.)

The house was my dream come true. From the front we looked on to the canal, at the back we had views over the Chilterns. We kept chickens, which I trained to come and jump on boxes, just for the fun of it. We also bottle-reared two goats, but they were eventually rehomed at a children's pet area because they followed us around and didn't like being left – they were worse than the dogs.

There was a sad (for me) but inevitable moment when my beloved baby sister Simone left school and moved to Nottingham to train as a nurse. I felt almost as bereft without her around as she felt when I went to university when she was eight. But we're such a close family that she came home whenever there was a get-together. She worked as a nurse for a year, but like me she is a real doggy person, and through me she could see that it was possible to work full time with dogs.

So later I was thrilled when she joined Hearing Dogs as a placement officer. I was not her immediate boss, so there was no nepotism. If there had been, I would have kept her near to me! Instead she went to work in the northern centre, based at Goole in Yorkshire. It was while she was travelling back to see friends in Nottingham that she met her husband, John Brainch, and for a couple of years she based herself there while she covered the northern region.

They later moved back to Buckinghamshire when a job came up at the Hearing Dogs headquarters, near Princes Risborough. John told Simone on their second date that he didn't really like dogs, and she very nearly walked out there and then. But he has been converted, thankfully: I don't think you'd last very long in this family unless you like dogs!

I loved my work at Hearing Dogs, but I found it hard to close my eyes to what was happening in the wider world of dog training. I really disliked the techniques being used in many training classes, and it distressed me to see people in the street and in parks trying to dominate their dogs. It was a combination of my background in psychology, my work training a rat and my experience at Hearing Dogs that convinced me this was wrong, and that using stimuli and rewards was a much better route to getting a dog to do what you want.

I read about the training of dolphins, and although I am always concerned about the way animals like these are held captive in unsuitable conditions, it was clear they were not being trained by domination. There were no trainers in the water with them, hitting them or frightening them: they were responding to the stimulus of the whistle or the clicker, which brought them a reward. My feelings about dog training, which I'd held for many years, grew stronger, to the extent that I came to believe we were abusing our relationship with the most sensitive and caring animal in our lives. Those people yelling at their dogs in the park would instinctively know that you can't train a chicken or a fish by shouting at it. You wouldn't house-train a chicken by rubbing its beak in its own mess, any more than you would do that with a human baby.

If you smack a dog's nose, or yank on a choke chain, the dog will learn because ultimately dogs are good at learning. But why do it this way? To get the best out of an animal you have to try to see the world through its eyes, and then bring learning theory in on top of that. Our domesticated dogs have been bred for centuries to be biddable, to want to do what's right for us. They are constantly searching our faces to find out what we want, and by giving them confused messages they do what they think is right, then get punished if they get it wrong.

Yes, by dominating a dog you can make it behave. But what a shame for the relationship: the close companionship we can have with our dogs is the biggest bonus these gentler methods of training bring. I found I was becoming more and more passionate about this. And I was also still thinking about Gill's story, and others that I read about in newspapers from time to time of dogs spontaneously alerting their owners to health dangers.

These dogs were confident enough to tell their owners something: a terrified and bullied dog would never dare to do that.

Clicker training, which is the method I use, was first invented in the late 1940s, but it didn't catch on in Britain until the late eighties and early nineties. It involves using a clicker with a sharp sound to tell a dog (or any other animal) when it has done the right thing, and the click is followed by a reward, and therefore the click is a 'conditioned reinforcer'. It is a consistent, easy-to-hear sound, and works much better than simply saying 'yes' or 'good boy'. It is incredibly powerful because it identifies the exact point where the dog has made the right decision, and, more importantly, by using it I can read the dog's thought processes.

There is research evidence that dogs learn 50 per cent faster using the clicker method. It can be used with very young puppies, and it takes away stress from the owner/trainer. It's possible to use other methods, but the clicker has been proven to be the best, and is the one we use now that we train medical assistance dogs and cancer-detection dogs.

My professional and personal interest in dog training led to me applying for membership of a relatively new organisation, the Association of Pet Behaviour Counsellors, which was established to try to regulate trainers and canine behaviourists, and discourage those who had no qualifications but set themselves up as experts. The APBC aims are to maintain very high professional standards among canine behaviourists, and to promote the profession so that anyone using a trainer will look for their APBC accreditation. They give support to trainers, and also provide a forum for us all to exchange ideas and theories about pet behaviour.

To become a member of the APBC I had to produce a portfolio of my work, and evidence that I had a degree in a subject that was appropriate. Case studies were needed, and naturally I couldn't use my own dogs. Perhaps the most common problem I had to deal with, and it is still today the most common problem for pet dogs, is separation anxiety. We've bred dogs, which are essentially pack animals, to be part of our group, in our lives. Then we go out to work and leave one dog alone for eight or nine hours, and we wonder why it is so distressed and why its behaviour is destructive.

When anyone buys a dog they should look closely at what that dog has been bred for. Collies, for example, are bred to be sheepdogs, and this is one area where instinctive prey-drive behaviour is used. The chain starts with eye stalking, when they stop and stare, followed by hunting their prey, and ending with grabbing, biting and killing. Obviously, the final stages of the chain have been bred out, which means they are fantastic at rounding up sheep, using the first steps of the chain, without normally touching them.

So it is hardly surprising that the collie, which has amazing eye-stalk skills, incredible hearing and sight – he can hear the shepherd's whistle from three fields away in a howling gale on the Yorkshire Dales – and is very aroused by movement, doesn't respond well to being shut in a London flat all day, and then develops the urge to chase traffic.

Other dogs, like beagles who were bred to hunt foxes, don't have the first part of the chain – they don't do eye stalk – but as a pack they have the end part, the hunting, biting and killing elements. So the owners should not be surprised when a solitary beagle, living in a family home, takes off in pursuit of a deer or a rabbit and does not return when called.

Aggression is the other main reason I am called in to help with a pet dog, often at the point where the dog is about to be put down. In eight out of ten cases it is possible to turn an aggressive dog round: the main reason for aggression is that the dog is confused and has never developed good impulse control. Owners fail to read the warning signs that their dog is uncomfortable and likely to become aggressive if not helped to deal with the situation. Sadly, I accept that there are a small number of dogs that will always show aggression, either because they come from a breed that has over many years been genetically selected for aggression, or because they have had a very poor start in life.

I was thrilled when the executive of the APBC unanimously voted for me to become a full member in 1991 (and years later, in 2009, I was delighted to become an

Honorary Life Member). It was exhilarating for me to meet so many other people who shared my philosophy and understanding of the work. I went to conferences and seminars, and was passionately involved with the association.

I loved the fact that everyone at the APBC wanted to train dogs by reward, not by domination. There is an area, however, where I disagree with some members, and they are the ones who believe you should never tell off a dog, that they should only learn by positive experience. They don't believe you should ever use the word 'no' to a dog but, as I said about teaching impulse control, I believe that there are times when dogs need to understand that behaviour has consequences.

Of course, horrible stuff like electric collars, kicking, choke chains and bullying are absolutely out. But when a dog is doing something you do not want him to do, I would say 'no'. A few words of disapproval are often all it takes (dogs are brilliant at reading how we feel, and they want to please us). Then he gets a reward when he does it right, and he feels happy and wants to do it that way again.

Some things we train dogs for are neutral tasks. For example, if I'm training a dog to sit, when he does it, he gets a reward. It's easy. But if I'm training a dog that has been bred and worked as a gun dog not to chase rabbits when we are out for a walk, that's very different. The dog wants to chase, but he has to be taught to discriminate when it is right to behave in this way and when it is wrong. A lot of trainers believe this is impossible, and simply avoid putting their dogs in those situations.

But this is where the building blocks come in. You have to train a non-aroused dog before you can expect it to behave the way you want when it is aroused. Most people ask a dog to do something in a situation where there are distractions, before they've established the behaviour in an environment without distractions.

Some owners don't understand why a dog that is highly motivated by food (it will learn to sit, and to bring back a tennis ball, for the reward of a biscuit) won't come back for a biscuit when it is on the scent of a rabbit. The rabbit chase impulse is so strong that a biscuit is meaningless – it doesn't even see the biscuit – and if the owner shouts, the dog is so intensely focused on the rabbit that it hears the shout as a faint whisper.

So the reinforcers for good behaviour vary hugely, according to the situation. If I were training a dog not to chase rabbits, I would start training in an area where he would not encounter a rabbit. Then I'd use a rabbit dummy, covered in real rabbit fur, and every time I called the dog off a real rabbit, I'd throw the dummy for him several times as a reward. That would redirect his energy and give him the same sense of arousal. It's important to find a diversion, a release for that pent-up energy. Shouting and punishing the dog just makes him more frustrated and leads to worse problems.

Like humans, different dogs put different values on things, and you have to learn to read your dog. Some dogs love food; some love a cuddle; some want toys; some are very possessive about their toys, bones or chews; some dogs are mortified if they are told off and a look of disapproval is all it takes to make them behave. Understanding their values is key to training them, and I don't recommend using their highest reward for simple tasks like learning to sit: yes, reward them, but keep the reward they value the most for a difficult task like, say, not chasing a rabbit.

One of the worst areas of dog training, Andy and I both felt, was with gun dogs, where highly intelligent dogs were trained to do amazing work finding and retrieving, but were frequently bullied into submission and obedience by harsh training. We wanted to prove that dogs could perform just as well if trained our way, by reward and co-operation, and that's what we set out to do.

I love seeing gun dogs working at the height of their powers: moving fast, searching by odour, sniffing the wind, all their instincts heightened. There are times in gun-dog work where the dog knows better than you do. One of the tasks they are tested on is retrieving canvas dummies, which are launched into the air and land as far as two fields away, and the job of the handler is to hold the mark, which means remembering where the dummy fell, looking away from it, and being able to look back at the same spot. The dog follows the handler's gaze.

The old boys in gun-dog training are tough, and they often use methods that I regard as brutal. I've been to seminars where top trainers have advocated pinning a dog down, kicking it so badly it could scarcely walk, to make it do the right thing. I've seen this in practice, and it made me physically sick. The trainers would say the dog had to be taught to do what it was told, but I knew there was another way to do this.

I got into gun-dog training mainly because I wanted to make a difference, but also because I love the sight of a humanely treated dog working at full stretch and using all its natural instincts. It is wonderful to see, and I soon had Ruffles working at a high level. Minstrel, too, would work, but I was never quite sure how good he would be . . .

Ruffles was so good that when I didn't have time to play with him he'd devise his own game. If there was a piece of paper in the garden he would wait for the wind to blow it, then he would practise his own internal control, doing 'Sit' and 'Stay' until the paper had blown further away, then he would release himself to chase it. It was as if an invisible person was controlling him. If there was no wind, he'd pat it to make it move. It was very funny watching him.

Andy is a very good trainer, and he and I would trundle off together and compete with our dogs. You have to have really good timing to be a good gun-dog trainer, catching the dog before it goes wrong. The better you predict what it will do, the easier you can train it.

Dill is another of my wonder dogs, who came into my life after Ruffles died. He was bred by a gun-dog trainer I met at a competition, a lovely farmer called Charles Morris who ran a traditional farm in the Midlands, with shire horses and Gloucester Old Spot pigs. He seemed to belong in a long-ago world, as if he didn't quite fit in the modern age. Sadly, he later died from a heart attack when he was throwing out hay for his animals, a shock to many who knew him because he looked so fit. His funeral, which Andy and I went to, was an appropriately eccentric event. We took time off work to go, and as usual we were cutting it fine with the time. As we came off the M42 on to a dual carriageway, we found ourselves in a queue of slow-moving traffic and we were getting anxious about whether we would make it in time. After a while, we could see that the problem was a vehicle ahead of us that was going very slowly and holding up the traffic, but we could see that cars were eventually getting round it. It was only when we were close that we realised that ahead of us were two beautiful shire horses pulling a farm cart, on which sat the coffin of Charles. We were actually in the funeral procession, and it seemed right that his last journey should be behind the horses he loved so much.

I met Charles when he was judging a gun-dog competition, and he mentioned that he had a litter of cocker spaniel puppies. I went to see them and Dill, whose kennel name was Whitlocks Nymph, looked at me with this intense little face, staring me in the eye, as if at that very early age he had decided I was the one, and he wanted to know exactly what I wanted from him.

Ever since I was a child and watched the animation series *The Adventures of Parsley the Lion*, I wanted a dog called Dill, named after the character in the series who is hyperactive and mischievous. As soon as I met this little puppy I thought: 'You are my Dill.'

He learned his own name after only two or three repetitions – I think Minstrel needed more than a hundred! At eight weeks old I was doing gun-dog training with him. Soon afterwards, he'd sit and watch me, with an entire field between us, and never allow himself to be distracted. He won his first gun-dog puppy test at ten months old.

Dill was a remarkable gun dog. He could do anything, working like there was a mini computer in his head. I ran him against all the top, traditionally trained gun dogs, and he was right up there with the very best. He was very obedient, and in competition we would hold each other's gaze.

I also trained him to be a demonstration dog at Hearing Dogs. Other trainers told me I wouldn't be able to train him to do both, and I should decide what I wanted from him. Training for Hearing Dogs means responding to outside stimuli, like a doorbell, whereas gun-dog training relies on commands from the handler, so they are different skills.

I thought: 'Why can't a dog take on two different concepts?'

Dill proved I was right, lapping it all up, easily separating the two in his own head. He went on eventually to win the title Dog Brain of Britain, in a competition run by *Dogs Today* magazine, and was presented with a large medal and his own little mortar board. This resulted in lots of publicity, with Dill and me appearing on television programmes and at shows. Again, I conquered my shyness by concentrating entirely on Dill, and getting the best from him. To win the competition I trained him to find missing keys, even if they were in a pocket inside a washing machine. He could open the door of the machine and sniff them out. He was in great demand, appearing in a week of appeals for *GMTV* for their Get Up and Give Appeal, answering the phone as if dealing with a caller.

Yet at the same time he was excelling at gun-dog competitions. His retrieving was spot on; he was a real hunter. There are three types of retrieving that gun dogs are tested for: one where they see the mark, one where they don't but go on directions from the handler and then scent, and the third is a memory retrieve, where other things intervene between the mark being put out and the dog retrieving it. Dill was good at all of them but excelled at the memory retrieve: he could go through a whole hour of other things and still work out where the mark was.

I taught him not just to recognise from my hand positions where he should go, but also from my feet. Other dog trainers and judges were gobsmacked by him. I think they wondered how this woman who used such unusual training techniques had managed to get such amazing results.

I have a wonderful portrait of Dill done by a very good artist who has captured his soul: I've had other paintings of dogs that have missed the essence of that particular dog, and are simply portraits of a breed. But this one is very good, and was organised as a surprise present for me by Andy. There was only one problem: Andy gave the artist a photograph of Dill to work from, but in the picture he has a large card saying 'First Prize' in front of him, obscuring his feet. The artist asked Andy for a picture of Dill's feet but Andy could not find one, and instead gave her a picture of the feet of Pogle, another cocker spaniel.

When the picture was unveiled for me, I immediately said: 'Why has Dill got Pogle's feet?'

'Oh God, can you tell?' said Andy, who thought I would not notice. But I would have known Dill's feet anywhere. So it's a beautiful portrait, and it hangs in pride of place in my home, but it is definitely Dill with Pogle's feet, and it is an enormous credit to the artist that her work is so good I could recognise they were the wrong feet!

Dilly only really enjoyed working for me, and didn't work too well for Andy. But Andy trained Dill's daughter, Pippin, and she was also fantastic. We had other great dogs. I bought Tarka, a field spaniel, for Andy as a wedding present, and she went on to win more competitions than any other dog we had. Tarka was very bright and although Ruffles, who was still alive then, was leader of the pack, she soon worked out how to manipulate both him and Minstrel.

There's an ongoing debate about whether dogs show true insight, and although plenty of people like me believe that they do, it is very hard to prove. Tarka, I would argue, used insight when she demonstrated how to steal bones from both Minstrel, the amiable buffoon, and Ruffles, an altogether greater challenge. She played with Minstrel, flirting and teasing him, turning her tail towards him in a gesture that implied she wanted to be mated. He'd leave his bone to play with her, and then she would swoop and nick it. Poor old Minstrel would look puzzled, as if to say: 'How did that happen?'

But Tarka was clever enough to know that Ruffles wouldn't fall for this trick. She observed that he was a great guard dog, barking at any unexpected visitors. So she went to the front door and barked excitedly, as if there were someone there, and Ruffles would charge out to defend his territory. Tarka would then slip away and help herself to his neglected bone. The first time she did this, it worked, so she did it again.

I can never prove that she didn't work out how to do this by trial and error, rather than by reasoning and insight. But I'm sure in my own mind. She was also clever enough to tell us when something was amiss with the other dogs, once alerting us to one of the dogs digging a giant hole in the garden, and on another occasion that one of them had managed to get his nose into a bag of food. She even told us that the puppies had escaped, and once when one new puppy trotted off on his own down the footpath, she came to us and made such a fuss that we checked and discovered he was missing. She clearly knew what was right and wrong in our eyes, and decided on each occasion to tell us.

Tarka's intelligent behaviour was another seed for my belief that we were not harnessing the incredible power dogs had to improve our lives. She was able to communicate with us in a very subtle way, and had an instinctive feel for when we needed to know something. Surely this ability and willingness to help could be applied in other ways. I'm not saying that, as I watched her, I had any premonition about my future work training dogs to detect cancer, but she reinforced my view that we were not tapping the knowledge and understanding of dogs fully.

We bred dogs, having three litters in all, the first from Dill's half-sister Retty. I was really worried when she began to give birth – it felt like a huge responsibility, but thankfully it went very well. She had five puppies, and it was hard parting with them. Very recently, I had an email from someone who took one of them, to say his dog died after a long and extremely happy life, and thanking us for breeding him.

We had another litter from Retty's daughter, but breeding was very time-consuming, with all the socialising and house-training involved, then the sadness of parting with them. Dill fathered several litters of puppies for other breeders, but for some reason in most cases he didn't throw his looks or character into the puppies.

With all our dogs I used the same training methods that had worked so well with Dill and his predecessors. But they still hadn't caught on fully in the wider dog-training community. I went to a competition in Scotland once, running a dog called Oak who was a half-brother to Dill. I was with a top Labrador trainer, who saw me using clicker training with Oak.

'Why are you doing that?'

'It's how he knows he has done something right. That's how I taught him.'

'Do you know how I train mine? When they don't do it right I give them a bollocking.'

He was getting great results, and his method clearly works. But I would argue that his dog was not as confident and happy as my dogs, and that by adopting the old master/slave attitude he was missing out on the most rewarding part of the relationship.

Oak was a good little dog, and was shaping up very well in gun-dog trials. I was offered a lot of money for him by a friend who wanted a gun dog, and I accepted. He went on to become an excellent gun dog, and I missed him terribly because he had a lovely temperament, but at the time we needed the money and it was a very good offer. I still wish I'd kept him. The moment he was gone, I felt I had made a mistake.

It was while we were at Hearing Dogs that I went to Italy to advise on dog training at the San Patrignano community, a large drug rehabilitation centre near Rimini. It was founded in 1978 by an Italian entrepreneur from a wealthy background, who decided to throw open his farm to any drug addicts who agreed to take part in a four-year programme. It's completely free, relying on public donations and the family trust for funding, and it operates as a community in which all the residents share the chores and are trained in a whole range of life skills. Money is also raised by selling cheese, furniture and other goods made by the residents, plus pedigree puppies that they breed there.

When addicts join the community, they go cold turkey, which has caused controversy in the past. But the vast majority of them stick it and when they leave after four years, 70 per cent remain clean, which is a very high percentage for a rehab programme. Newcomers are assessed and then taught skills in areas that suit their natural interests.

I was invited to teach some dog trainers so that they could, in turn, teach others to train dogs. Andy came with me and we were picked up at the airport by a group of tough-looking men. I caught myself thinking, 'They look like drug addicts,' before I remembered that this was exactly what they were prior to joining the community.

When I arrived, I was immediately shown a very formal demonstration of their dog training, which involved a lot of yanking and pushing the dogs around. I was seated with three or four of the top people running the community, and I watched as the first three trainers demonstrated with their dogs, which behaved very well. The next man had a spaniel, the breed I know so well from Ruffles. The dog was defensive and unco-operative, and the man was clearly very unhappy because he felt he was failing. I could see the dog was saying to him: 'If you do that again, I'll bite you.' The dog was showing all the classic signs of frustrated aggression, as was the handler, who was failing in front of everyone.

I asked if we could stop the demonstration so that I could help. The organisers looked nonplussed, but they agreed. I went to the man and his dog and began to show him what he needed to do, using eye contact and rewards, not all the pushing and shoving he had been doing. The dog started to perform, and the guy who was handling it began to do it himself, without my help.

Afterwards he came to me and said, through my interpreter: 'Thank you. I always fail at everything, but I want to work with dogs. I will never forget the kindness you showed me today.'

I didn't tell him that I did it for the dog's sake ...

We spent two weeks there. We all ate together in a communal dining room, doors were never locked, and I had a 'buddy' assigned to me who went everywhere with me: it's part of the rehab process, and visitors are expected to observe the same rules as the residents. Everything I saw at San Patrignano was inspirational in terms of helping people. In the dog-training section where I worked, my message was: if you mutually respect each other, which is the ethos of the community, you must also respect dogs.

I gave up gun-dog trialling in about 2001. It slowly dawned on me that the higher you get in the competition world, the more the dogs are regarded as commodities. The stakes become ever higher. I'd set out to prove that it was possible to train dogs humanely, but now I found myself getting stressed because of all the competing I was doing. We also needed a lot of dogs to compete at such high levels: at one point Andy and I had twelve dogs living with us, which is far too many. You begin to lose sight of them as individuals, and you can't give each of them what they need.

I used to take on dogs that had been badly trained, and I enjoyed rehabilitating them and passing them on either as family pets or to work as gun dogs. Inevitably, though, I could never have the same close relationship with all these dogs as I did with the two or three really special ones.

Another reason we gave up gun-dog competitions is because we both became very interested in horses as I had been all my life: I had ponies when I was young and always loved the feeling of being on horseback. We bought two horses and we started competing with them at weekends, doing some showjumping, lots of cross-country and sponsored rides. We had no room at the cottage to stable the horses, so we kept them at livery, which was very expensive, and ultimately prompted our move away from the home we loved. At the time, Andy and I were also trying for a family, but sadly I was never able to get pregnant.

I didn't know it then, but I was about to start on the biggest, most exciting phase of my life. Before that, though, I'd like to tell you about one very special dog, who was my companion through the darkest times of my life, and who taught me so much.

CHAPTER FOUR

Woody

Asking me to choose the most special of all my dogs is like asking a mother to name her favourite child: I really can't. But if I were forced to choose, perhaps the strongest contender would be Woody. No, he wasn't a well-trained obedience dog. No, he never took part in gun-dog trials. No, if he were alive now I wouldn't be able to use him in the specialist work of Medical Detection Dogs.

But, yes, he was the most amazing, wonderful, awe-inspiring, determined little character I have ever met, a dog who defied everything to live a full and happy life. He was brave, affectionate and an inspiration to everyone who met him. He was also mischievous, full of fun, and up for anything the other dogs were doing – which was, in itself, incredible.

Woody was born after I mated Dill with a friend's bitch, a field-trial champion. Dill loved hunting, but was not a field-trial expert, so this looked like a good match, and I was all set to choose one of the puppies when the litter arrived. The breeder was an established gun-dog breeder, feeding his working dogs on tripe which he bought from a local farmer.

I went to see the puppies soon after birth, and was delighted to see that this was one litter where Dill had clearly left his stamp. With the whole litter to pick from, I fixed on a little fella who looked like a replica Dill, with the same chocolate colouring, and decided I would call him Woody. I loved the novels of Thomas Hardy, and often chose names for dogs from them – Retty, Izzy. But I couldn't hit on a suitable name for this little fella, until I thought of *The Woodlanders*. As his kennel name was Gamegoer Woodman, it seemed appropriate. Lots of people assumed he was named after the character in the film *Toy Story*, especially as my sister Simone had a cocker we rescued from the brink of death and which she called Buzz, but that was just a coincidence.

I went to visit my little pup every week, a round trip of about sixty miles, because like all puppies he needed to stay with his mother for seven or eight weeks. It was on my third visit, when he was just five weeks old, that I noticed he was looking weak and wobbly on his legs.

'What's the matter?' I asked the breeder.

'He's gone a bit gimpy, I don't know why.'

I went back a couple of days later and he was much worse, and had lost the use of his back legs. The mother, like many working dogs, fed her puppies standing up, and it was obvious this little chap couldn't reach her teats, and was not doing well among his more robust brothers and sisters.

He was clearly hungry. The breeder would lob treats into the pen and the puppy would squirm across like a little worm, his back legs completely useless.

'Can I take him to my vet?' I asked the breeder.

'You can if you like,' he shrugged. 'But I doubt there's anything he can do. You can choose yourself another puppy.'

I scooped up Woody and took him to Colin Price, who put him on the table with a look on his face that said, 'Here's Claire, with another disaster ...'

He didn't know what was wrong, but put Woody on antibiotics, telling me that he may come round, and to bring him back in two days.

I took Woody back to his mum, but on the way I had an inspiration.

'I've got a bitch, Jasmine, who has just had puppies, only three, so she's got spare milk, and she feeds them lying down. Would you mind if I took Woody to see if she will feed him?' I asked the breeder.

He was happy to let me have the little problem puppy. Jasmine allowed him to feed without a fuss, but she didn't take to him: she didn't do any other mothering, and wouldn't let him snuggle up with her other pups. She didn't accept him, but allowed him to suckle, which at least meant he was getting enough food.

Woody's back legs remained paralysed, but he could scuttle across the floor, dragging them behind him. I took over the role of mum to him, carrying him around with me, fastened into my fleece with his little head poking out of the top. He slept on my pillow at night. He was bright as a button, with alert eyes following everything. But his paralysis was getting worse: his left front leg was partially affected and he was clearly growing weaker; his tail was paralysed and he couldn't wag it. One of his eyes was twitching and starting to close, a sign that the paralysis was creeping towards it.

Finally I reconciled myself to putting him out of his suffering, and booked what I thought was going to be his last appointment at the vet's. He was on the table in the surgery and Colin and I looked at each other, neither of us relishing what was going to happen.

'Is there nothing else you can do?'

Colin shook his head, sadly. I was holding Woody, who was gazing at me with his big, trusting eyes.

'Wait. It's a long shot, but there may be something,' Colin suddenly said. 'It's very unlikely. But there is a new disease in cattle that's been identified in the last few years, called neospora. It causes paralysis and internal damage. It can happen in dogs, but it's very rare and I've never seen it in a dog.'

Neospora is a neuromuscular disease that was first identified in dogs in Norway, more than ten years earlier, but it had been misdiagnosed for some years and was only recently becoming a risk for dogs in the UK. Colin carried out a blood test to be sent to a laboratory for confirmation that Woody had neospora, but the little chap was so ill that we both agreed treatment should start even before the condition was confirmed, as it wasn't looking good for him. Besides, it sounded possible, and it was easy to see how he had contracted it: his mother had been eating uncooked tripe from a farm. The most common way for dogs to pick up neospora is from eating the tissue of infected cattle, and there is a vicious circle because the faeces of dogs with neospora are what spread the disease in cows.

I felt so relieved that there was another possibility to save little Woody.

Colin started him on a powerful drug regime, but it seemed that perhaps it was too late. Woody languished in his basket, with hardly the energy to lift his head, getting weaker and weaker. I still carried him around with me, but his spark seemed to have dimmed. Eventually, I began to feel it was wrong to prolong his life. I knew, having read up about neospora, that the best we could hope for was to stop the creeping paralysis, and that he would never get the use of his hind legs back.

'The prognosis is poor in puppies if the disease has progressed to hind limb paresis, with atrophied, rigid limbs,' I read in one of my veterinary books.

But I determined to give him the best shot, and at least complete the course of drugs. Thank goodness I did, because three days later he looked up at me from his bed and wagged his funny little tail, weakly. I could hardly believe it, and to this day I have no idea how or why the nerves in his tail started to work again, but it was the clearest sign he could give that he had turned a corner, and the future was hopeful. His joy in life was back, and he began to wriggle across the floor again to join in any fun the other dogs were having.

Colin Price was almost as thrilled as I was, but he warned me that one of the consequences of neospora is that Woody's heart might be damaged and could give out at any time, and that he would probably die suddenly, and young. He said he could die in the night, and I would find him dead in the morning. He was right to tell me, but I put that thought aside: my big project now was to get Woody up on to his feet, and I was determined to do it. As far as he was concerned, I was his mum, a role I played for the rest of his life. He had a high-pitched scream that he used whenever he needed me, a puppy scream that other dogs grow out of as they get older. It was always a signal to me that Woody was in trouble, probably with his paralysed legs trapped somewhere.

I started intensive physiotherapy with him, massaging his atrophied back legs. He had some residual feeling in them: he could tell when I was touching his feet. But they had no power or strength in them. I was determined to help him stand but it was a very long, difficult road. He was so small that I could put him in our bath, and do swimming therapy with him there. I devoted all my spare time to him, and within two weeks there was an amazing moment when he managed to get to his feet, just for a few seconds, using his two back legs together as one.

By this time his tail was wagging so much that it only stopped when he was asleep: this was a clear sign that he was improving.

I used clicker training, and my goal was to teach him control of his legs, and to take short steps. I watched him carefully, and began to teach him to recognise any slight feelings in the nerve endings. We made great progress. It was not a miracle: both his back legs remained paralysed and always worked as one, and it was very hard teaching him to co-ordinate them with his front legs. He would fall over, and then revert to dragging his legs behind him. He could only walk in a straight line, flopping his rear end to the floor if he needed to turn. Could I do anything more for him? He was a huge challenge to my dog-training theories and abilities.

Having got him walking in his own fashion, my aim was to teach him to turn without falling over. I taught him to use his partially paralysed front foot as a pedal, patiently showing him for days how he could turn left or right if he swung round on his good leg. It took weeks, but the rewards were immense. He came on in leaps and bounds. His strange gait became known as Woody's Amazing Clicker Walking. He could never run as fast or as long as my other dogs, but he could do an astonishing amount of things. He couldn't climb steps: I always carried him upstairs to bed, where he continued for the rest of his life to sleep snuggled up to me. He always knew he was special.

He accepted his limitations. He would watch the other dogs going up and down the stairs, but he didn't complain about it. Outside, if we came to steps in front of a building, he would look to the left and right, searching for the ramp that is often there for disabled people – and, as far as Woody was concerned, for disabled dogs. He loved our training sessions, and learned to sit on his damaged hindquarters, turn, and even do a small jump.

A couple of years later I was at a conference and a chap introduced himself to me, telling me he was a vet. He asked if Woody had suffered from neospora, and shook his head in wonder when I said he had.

'That dog of yours shouldn't be able to walk, but he looks almost normal. It's incredible. How did you do it?'

I learned a huge amount from Woody, more than from any other dog I have owned. But I don't take credit for his amazing recovery: I may have taught him what to do, but the guts and determination that got him up and about was his, and his alone.

After Colin's warning that he could die at any time, I treated every day as a bonus. And he lived every day as though it might be his last, throwing himself into any action that was going with the other dogs. When I took them for walks I had to lift him out of the boot of the car, but after that he was after them as fast as his damaged legs would carry him. He even tried to cock his leg, but in the end he decided it was easier not to bother, unless he was trying to impress another dog, when he would find a nearby tree to prop his leg against and wee like a male dog.

When I took all the dogs out for a walk, I always kept an eye out for when he was getting tired. Then I would carry him under my arm, or put him in a rucksack on my back, his little face poking out and his eyes darting to make sure he missed nothing. When he wanted to get down to join the other dogs he wriggled to get my attention.

One of my favourite walks was up Ivinghoe Beacon, a prominent hill in a National Trust-owned swathe of the Chiltern Hills. It is famously steep, so I always carried Woody for the first half of the climb, until I was red in the face and happy to give in to his demands to be put down. I also wanted to carry him on the way down because of the gradient. I was very worried that he would slip and hurt himself.

But Woody soon found his own way down, which he loved: he slid, going from side to side like a skier doing a slalom course. I was terrified for him, but he wagged his tail and loved every second of it, getting down almost as fast as the other dogs, then staggering to his wonky feet and looking back at me as if to say: 'Come on, slow coach.'

When I went swimming with my dogs during a week-end break in Dorset, Woody insisted on joining Tangle and Daisy in the sea with me. It's amazing that he could swim at all, but I was worried about him because I knew he would tire and get cold. But when I took him out of the water to a friend on the beach, he soon wriggled free and jumped back in with me.

I confess he was spoilt. I could never tell Woody off; he had such a cheeky face and the bond between us was so great. I always knew instantly when he felt unwell, as I do with all the special dogs I have a really close bond with. I could feel in his body the change in his energy.

He knew how to play up to other people, who were always fascinated by him. He'd tilt his head in a comical way, his tail wagging frantically, and they'd say, 'Oh, look at that little disabled dog . . .' Then they'd bend down to stroke him and any piece of food they might be holding would disappear in a trice. He had enough spring in his legs to be able to grab a sandwich when he fancied one.

He loved his food, probably because for those first important days of his life he was starved when he couldn't feed from his mother. He was also a real thief, though it took me a while to realise that this little, disabled dog was quite able, when he chose, to get up to the kitchen work-tops and steal food I left out.

When I acquired Daisy – another of my very special dogs – I was upset to think that she was turning into a thief. I'd come into the kitchen and the food would have disappeared, even though I'd pushed it to the back of the worktop.

'Daisy, you naughty girl!' I'd say, while Woody looked on with big eyes, quite happy for Daisy to get the blame.

Not liking a cross mum, Daisy would look really abashed and guilty, while Woody wagged his tail happily, which I foolishly took as confirmation that she was the culprit.

'It looks as if Daisy is going to be a bloomin' thief,' I said to Andy. 'I'm going to set her up and watch what she does.'

I left a plate of biscuits out, and hid in the next room to watch. Who did I catch? Not Daisy, who could easily have stolen the biscuits, but Woody, who with his damaged legs should not have been able to get near. He had learned that if he took a run up and launched himself at the kitchen unit, he could push his body up the cupboards with his front legs and quickly grab with his mouth what was left on top.

So I should have known better when another incident occurred on a break in a caravan in Dorset. My friend and I had bought two enormous Cornish pasties, spending ages choosing the flavours in a shop dedicated just to making them. On the drive back to the caravan we were salivating at the thought of them, the tempting smell filling the car. I put them on the worktop in the caravan kitchen area, and then got caught up talking to someone at the site water tap. The other dogs were still in the boot of the car, but I'd taken Woody into the caravan first.

Opening the door when I got back, Woody was sitting there like a little pot-bellied pig, with just a piece of crust and some paper to show for our lunch. I'll swear he was grinning at me. He'd eaten both enormous pasties and, because it was too far to go back to the pastie shop, we had to make do with some greasy chips from the local chippie.

This wasn't the last time he disgraced himself. When he was really old we were out walking when I saw an old couple sitting on a bench with their picnic in a bag at their feet.

'Pick up your bag!' I shouted, as Woody set off on a mission towards them.

They were so busy going 'Awww, look at this poor little doggy . . .' that they took no notice of my warning, and within no time Woody was rifling among their sandwiches and biscuits.

He was no pushover for the other dogs. When Tangle arrived, as a tiny puppy, three years before Daisy, Woody was very quick to tell him who was boss. He was completely in control, no matter how big and fit another dog was. I've observed over the years that the boss of a pack of dogs is rarely the strongest, but always the brightest and one with a great deal of energy. Ruffles was the boss until he died, then Dill took over, then Woody. It was astonishing to see this small, crippled dog running seven or eight others, all of them totally respectful towards him. They could easily have dominated him physically: he was so fragile that if you knocked into him he went down like a skittle.

The way a pack works, he was supported by dogs lower down the pack who worked together to keep him in charge: it's fascinating watching how the top dog maintains his position. I see it with my chickens, it works the same way. There's rarely any aggression: the leader maintains the pack serenely, by the force of their personality. In Woody's case, the other dogs knew he was in a strong coalition with me, and that it was not worth trying to take Woody on.

Despite Colin's warning about his life expectancy, my brave little Woody lived until he was fourteen and a half. I saved his life when he was tiny, and he thanked me every day with his devotion and enthusiasm. He came to work with me every day, shadowing me until the very end. He gave me constant, unquestioning love at all times. He was as brave as any warrior, and he, above all, gave me the courage to pull my own life around when things were bleak for me. When he died, in my arms, I was devastated, even though I knew he had far exceeded his projected lifespan, and he was elderly and very frail. My only consolation was knowing that nothing could ever harm him now. He was safe forever.

Three days after he died, I had a very powerful dream. I was walking along a path and I suddenly stopped as Woody came running towards me. It was a young Woody, full of life, but definitely him with his limping back legs. He ran up to me and looked at me in the way he did when he wanted me to pick him up. I scooped him into my arms and held him close, and we looked deep into each other's eyes. I could smell him, that little Woody Wood Chips smell that was so familiar. Then, after what seemed like quite a while, he gave the little wriggle that signalled he wanted to be put down. I put him on the ground and he looked back at me, wagging his tail the way he always wagged it. Then he ran off down the path. He stopped and looked back at me twice, and then he was gone.

I woke up and I could still smell him, still feel the weight of him in my arms. The pain was almost unbearable, I longed for him so much. I really hope that there is somewhere dogs go after death, somewhere where Ruffles is, and Dill can take care of Woody, who can boss Tangle . . .

Now, more calmly, I look back and remember Woody for his strength of character, cheerful disposition, and proof that immense obstacles can be overcome with determination and application, both his and mine. He gave me so much, and I believe he came into my life because I needed him as much as he needed me.

My beautiful Dill, Woody's father, died a few years earlier, when he was nearly twelve. He had put everything into his life, and he, too, had given everything to me. His death broke my heart, but ultimately I feel privileged to have owned a dog like him. The Guide Dogs for the Blind have a bank of frozen semen, and Dill is among the donors. One day, I hope I will breed from him with a nice cocker spaniel bitch, and end up with a puppy related to both him and Woody.

CHAPTER FIVE

The Maggot Man

'Did you hear it?' Gill was so excited that she almost danced up to me when I arrived at work.

'Hear what?'

'The radio. This doctor, he was talking about dogs detecting cancer. He's an expert on maggots being used to clean wounds.'

She could hardly catch her breath.

I'd been listening to CDs of my favourite soul music in the car, not tuned into the *Today* programme on Radio 4, so I shook my head as Gill rushed on.

'You'll never believe it . . . There was a doctor, talking about dogs being able to sniff out cancer. It's just what we've always said, but he's a *doctor*. He said he'd be interested in anyone who could train dogs and help him prove it. He's called John Church and he was saying all the things we say ...'

The fact that he'd appealed for a collaboration with dog trainers lit up my brain: this was what we needed, a proper scientific study into whether we could harness the amazing scent skills of dogs to detect cancer in a systematic way, not just by chance.

Gill rang the BBC and asked to be put in touch with the doctor. A polite switchboard operator took our details and promised to pass them on to him: understandably, she was not able to give us his number. Within hours, we had made contact with him. To our amazement, and in what John describes as 'wonderful serendipity', we discovered that he lived a twenty-minute drive away from Hearing Dogs, and he was free to come and meet up with me, Gill and Andy after work that same day. Somehow I knew, as soon as I met him, that we were destined to work together. I quickly outlined my past work with dogs, and he told me how he had first become interested in the whole area of research.

John is a retired orthopaedic surgeon whose life story is worthy of a book in itself. When he was a young doctor he spent four years working as a bush surgeon in Rwanda, during the first genocide of the Tutsi people, in the late fifties and early sixties. The Tutsi were being massacred by the Hutu, whose weapons were mainly spears and machetes. Some victims were left for dead but were later brought into the field hospitals alive, and, even under the stress of his awful workload, John noted that the survivors were those who had maggots in their wounds. The maggots were working away, eating the debris and putrefaction of the wounds, cleaning them better than any modern sterile treatment.

Later, back in the UK, John learned about the history of the use of maggots in medicine. In the Napoleonic

Wars, maggots were used to halt the spread of gangrene and septicaemia, and there is medical literature dating back nearly 400 years about their use. John combined his career and family life with his interest in maggots, and gave lectures on his experience in Rwanda. Through this he met an American doctor who was pioneering work with maggots, using them in a veterans' hospital to treat ulcers on the legs of elderly people, and this inspired John to collaborate with a consultant dermatologist in Oxford on the first use of maggots in this country in modern times, including building a maggot-breeding facility in his own garage. John treated the first thirty patients in Britain whose wounds were cleaned and cured by maggots after all other treatments had failed, and has collaborated in research to isolate the effective enzyme the maggots are producing.

It was another serendipitous event that led John on from maggots to his fascination in the ability of dogs to detect cancer. He gave a lecture on his maggot work to students at Westminster College, a further education college in London. He had recently read a letter in the *Lancet*, a medical journal, written by two dermatologists who had treated a woman for a malignant melanoma after her dog alerted her to a small mole. It was a story that completely echoed Gill's experience.

John mentioned it in his lecture to the students, using it as an example of the ways in which animals have superior senses, which, if harnessed, could be of great benefit to mankind. Later, over the dinner hosted by the college,

John sat opposite a young man who said: 'You must meet my father.'

He told how his father's skin cancer had been detected by a dog showing unusual interest in a patch of eczema on his leg, nudging it constantly. John subsequently spent four hours with the young man's father, and the story generated some media interest. Ultimately, John collected together thirty stories of dogs detecting cancer, including breast cancer as well as melanoma, and published them in a long letter to the *Lancet*.

The problem was that the stories were all anecdotal. In every case the dog had a good relationship with its master, so it was unclear if the alert to cancer would only happen in those circumstances, or if it could be used in a more general – and hugely beneficial – way. So that's how John came to make his Radio 4 appeal for anyone who felt they could train dogs for the work to get in touch.

When we met John, we talked for hours, exploring possible ways we could harness dogs' olfactory senses to prove what we all believed, and to convince a sceptical world. More importantly, how could we make practical use of it, and actually start saving lives by detecting cancer? For me, it was wonderful meeting a man with distinguished medical credentials who took the subject seriously, and had complete confidence that we would one day prove it.

His attitude, all the way through, has been to ignore the wall of scepticism we hit from the medical and scientific professions.

'Let's do it,' he said. 'What does it matter if we're wrong? What have we lost? And we won't be wrong.'

John was thrilled to meet Gill and hear her story, and Andy and I told him all about our work training gun dogs.

We knew the problems we faced. It was not simply a matter of training the dogs: I was reasonably sure we could do that, although detecting cancer odours was going to be much trickier than training dogs that are used to detect drugs, explosives or even human bodies in disaster areas. In all those cases, the dogs are trained with the material they are expected to find. A drug dog looking for heroin will be trained with samples of heroin: how on earth were we going to train dogs on samples of cancer? How were we going to persuade the medical profession to allow us to invade their clinical area? What sort of samples could we work on?

When we finally all went home, my head was buzzing. Andy was also very enthusiastic, but I was the one who was really taken by it, with a huge determination to get the project up and running. I hardly slept: my mind was going over and over the possible ways we could establish a trial to prove what we all believed. I knew this was going to be my main focus, that my work with Hearing Dogs was no longer enough for me, and for personal reasons I was no longer as fulfilled as I had been there.

This was the onset of a period of huge, personal unhappiness in my life, the start of a terrible time for me. But I did not know this then, and it is only today, with the benefit of hindsight, that I can see that the feeling of no longer being so tied to Hearing Dogs freed me to do the work that is by far the most important thing I have ever done.

At this time, Andy and I were taking our horses very seriously, and we were offered another one on loan. We knew that if we paid for three at livery it would cost £20,000 a year out of taxed income: we simply couldn't do it. We decided we needed to buy a place with enough land for us to keep the horses, so we sold our delightful canalside cottage and bought a one-bedroom semi near Quainton, Bucks. The house was far inferior, but it came with three fields and stables, and at that moment the horses were our driving force. We moved with our dogs: I had Dill, Woody, Tangle and Daisy, and Andy had Tarka, Reddle, Pippin and Retty.

The house move proved to be a disaster. Our new home was half of a farmhouse, and when the building was split the internal walls put up between the two halves were not thick. We could literally hear everything in the bedroom adjoining ours, even being able to make out conversations, and we were certainly aware of the rumbling snore next door that sounded as if it were in the same room.

It was very stressful. We only had one bedroom, so I couldn't escape to another room. I bitterly regretted our move, which we made because we were so ambitious with our horses. With hindsight, we should have turned down the third horse and reminded ourselves how much we loved our canalside cottage.

Even the horses were a problem: it is hard to look after three when you are working full time, and as we both had senior jobs at Hearing Dogs, it was always a problem if one of us had to miss work for a vet's visit.

I had risen from assistant trainer, to trainer, then head trainer, training manager and, by the time Andy and I had been married for ten years, I was operations director. Andy may have felt that my presence there restricted him: I was there before he was; I was a member of the APBC; I had driven the training forward. But on the other hand he was better at writing reports than I was, and enjoyed the public speaking, so he became technical director, doing admin, fundraising and being a very good spokesman for the charity.

Andy and I were always competitive, whether with dogs or horses. At the same time, we were both very proud of the other: if he was competing I felt a huge rush of pride when he won, and at the time I thought he felt the same about me.

Unfortunately, we became competitive in another way. When Tony Blunt, the founder and original CEO of Hearing Dogs, retired, an interim CEO was appointed. Tony was a doggy person, who understood what we were doing and was very supportive, always listening to me when I talked about the training, and giving me a free rein to get on with it my own way. The new CEO had a different approach, which didn't always chime with my way of doing things.

The change meant that my thrill at being part of the charity waned, and I stopped being enthusiastic about my job. The CEO made it clear that she did not intend to stay long, and Andy coveted her job, although there were those on the staff who felt it should rightly go to me. It was a very bad time, and looking back I probably should have left Hearing Dogs at this juncture.

But I didn't: I stuck it out, and the great benefit of this is that I was there when Gill heard John Church on the radio. So, looking back, everything was working for the best, and towards my future. But at the time it was tough, not helped by my feelings towards the new house.

Andy and I stayed in the house for two and half years, and I hated it all that time. I was never reconciled to losing the lovely home I had before. We looked into insulating the wall between the two houses, but it was not possible at a reasonable price and without massive disruption.

Andy decided to go for the chief executive job, and despite friends and colleagues urging me to apply, I said I would leave the field clear for him. Then a bombshell was dropped: if he got the CEO's job, I would not be able to continue working as operations director, and I would have to resign or step down to a lesser role. Much as I loved Andy, I couldn't help thinking: 'Hang on, I've worked really hard to get here.'

But I was still keen for him to succeed, and agreed that if he got the job I would step aside and become research director, with no staff under me, and no conflict of interest in the management line of command. Naturally, I felt hurt and pushed out.

Eventually, a new CEO was appointed, and it was not Andy: it was someone from outside the charity. Andy seemed angry, and blamed me, saying I had made it difficult for him. I admit I had not hidden my disappointment at potentially losing my job: I felt I had done so much for Hearing Dogs, setting up the training programme and procedures. So perhaps my barely concealed distress *was* the reason he failed to get the job, or maybe he simply wasn't thought to be the right man for it.

Andy seemed to me to be bitterly disappointed. He, too, had put his heart and soul into Hearing Dogs, and had an enormous amount invested in the charity emotionally.

We were both immature. I now know that Medical Detection Dogs will carry on very successfully without me one day. However much anyone does to set the ball rolling, the impetus carries on when that person moves on, and that is right. The organisation has its own validity, it is not a one-man band. But at the time, both Andy and I felt we had been kicked in the teeth, and we blamed each other.

But at this time John Church came into our lives, and for me the new project was the great challenge I needed. It was me who drove it, alongside John, and I took the lead on the dog-training side immediately. At our second meeting we discussed protocols, and John undertook to use his contacts at Bucks Healthcare NHS Trust to recruit help for us.

We knew that dogs have a hugely more efficient olfactory system than we humans do, mainly because they have twenty-five to thirty times more scent glands than we do, and that their sense of smell can be as much as ten million times more sensitive than ours. But how to harness it in complex research?

One of our first moves was to set up a small workshop to discuss the possibility of proper clinical trials. The CEO of Hearing Dogs agreed to let us run it on their premises at a weekend: they were very generous to us with use of their premises in those early days. We invited Michael McCulloch from California to talk to us. I'd read about his work using dogs to detect breast cancer from breath samples and he'd been getting some encouraging results. There was another researcher from Poland, Tadeusz Jezierski, who was also doing interesting work. They flew in at their own expense to share their experiences with us.

Dr Carolyn Willis, a senior researcher from the dermatology department of the Bucks Healthcare NHS Trust, also attended: it seemed logical to us all, at this stage, that if dogs could smell cancer it was more likely to be when the malignancy was close to the surface, in a mole or skin infection, as it was with most of the anecdotal cases.

From this beginning we had many more meetings with the trust, usually at their premises. Their support at this stage cannot be underestimated: without them the whole first trial would never have got off the ground. John's daughter Susannah, who is also a doctor, and Anthea Bransbury, a consultant dermatologist with the trust, both joined our discussions.

At our own expense, John, Susannah, Andy and I flew out to California to look at the work Michael McCulloch was doing. It was a very useful trip, if only to help us reject Michael's model of working from breath samples: today, we believe we will one day be able to use breath samples to detect some cancers, but it is still at a research and development level.

The most critical question was: what would we use to train the dogs with? We discounted using tumours that had been removed from cancer patients, because they would not be living tissue and the smell of chemical preservatives would mask the cancer scent. Skin samples from melanoma could be used, but only once: the minute they were defrosted and used, they would have to be discarded. Also, the ethical protocols for using tissue samples were very high. On top of that, how would we obtain healthy control samples to train the dogs with? We couldn't go round chopping lumps of skin off volunteers.

What we needed was a substance that contained the volatile organic compounds produced by malignant cells, without actually being itself cancerous. In other words, something that had been in contact with the tumour.

Urine now seems an obvious choice, as it clearly has contact with bladder cancer, but it took us a while to realise this. There were no precedents: we were working in completely new, unexplored, territory. Urine is also a relatively easy sample to obtain: giving a urine sample is non-invasive and something most people would happily agree to donate.

The difficulty is that there are other smells that urine can have, including those of other diseases, and sometimes blood in the sample. We needed to make sure that, despite these distractions, our dogs could single out cancer, a smell that we ourselves cannot detect.

It was a fraught time. We had this whole soup of smells in urine, and we were not, initially, even sure that cancer definitely had its own odour: we were going on instinct, reinforced by all the anecdotal and unproven stories of dogs alerting their owners to the disease. Nowadays it seems universally accepted that cancer cells have an odour, but it was all new ground then. It is easy to forget the struggle, the prejudice, and how completely at sea we were in finding a methodology. Night after night I lay awake: am I being really stupid trying to do this? Is it ever going to be possible?

Many of the traditional handlers I knew – police-dog handlers, gun-dog trainers and behaviour trainers – told me it would be impossible to train the dogs without giving them the original smell. When I said I was going to tackle it the other way round, they said it would be too difficult.

'How can you get a dog to detect an ingredient in something that has hundreds of ingredients?' I was constantly asked.

'By training them on something that hasn't got that one specific ingredient,' I replied. There was a lot of head shaking that went on.

We discussed the problem for hours, but in the end all agreed that urine samples were the best way forward. Carolyn and John set about getting samples for us, which was a lengthy process because medical protocols had to be followed. The NHS had to give ethical approval of the study, as we would be using NHS patients, and this took time. My problem, in the meantime, was could I train dogs to do the work, and what would I train them with?

We even tried appealing for cancer samples on a TV programme, but we were inundated with replies from patients who had already started treatment: we wanted samples from people in the brief window between diagnosis and treatment. It was clear that this was a very haphazard approach, and we had to wait until we could get proper samples through the trust.

My next dilemma was: which dogs should I choose?

The answer was simple: I put out an appeal to other dog trainers at Hearing Dogs, explaining that it would be time-consuming but ultimately satisfying work, and people came forward, volunteering their dogs and their own time to carry out the training. We decided to choose a complete cross-section of dogs of different breeds, different ages, different backgrounds, to see if any fared better than the others. Instinct told me that the breeds used as working dogs – spaniels and

Labradors – would be easier to train and would take to the work more naturally, but we were interested in testing this.

In fact, if we had followed that instinct, our first trial results would have been higher, and it is one of several things I would do differently if I were starting again. But we were working in a completely new field, there was no guidance we could follow: as the *British Medical Journal* report put it, there were 'no relevant peer-reviewed publications to refer to'. It is hard to believe now, but everything we did then was based on supposition, and we were taking a complete step into the unknown.

I was tough with the trainers, insisting that we all worked the same way. I explained that the stimulus has got to control the behaviour; there must be no preempting behaviours from the trainers. A couple of them pulled out after my first briefing session with them. One, who I met years later, said to me: 'I came to that first meeting and d'you know what? I thought you were totally mad, that you'd completely lost the plot.'

My evangelical zeal was clearly shining through ...

Dill, who was by now a really elderly dog, was my first guinea pig. I really just wanted to give myself confidence that the project would work. I knew that we could not use him in the main trial: his age, and his fame as Dog Brain of Britain, were against him. I soon had him sniffing out Earl Grey teabags when I hid them around the room, ignoring the PG Tips teabags, in order to get him used to the idea of being alert to something 'different' within a set of similar samples.

So with Dill's reassurance, it was time to start with our volunteers. We still did not have samples, but we decided to get them started on scent training, using teabags or fruit. Again, if I were starting the work now, I wouldn't do this: I'd be patient and wait for real samples. In retrospect it's possible to see that a urine sample could smell of Earl Grey tea if it came from a volunteer who had by coincidence been drinking the tea, which might confuse the dog if they'd been trained in this way. Nonetheless, we were impatient to get going, and I was keen to start scent discrimination trials.

We used clicker training for the dogs, and we worked at turning the dogs into the problem-solvers: we gave them the raw material, but they had to make the decisions. I felt as if all my work with dogs (and rats and other animals) had been leading to this.

I knew from training hearing dogs, who have to react to sound stimuli without any human intervention (because their deaf owners do not hear the sound), that the stimuli had to activate the behaviour. Working with odours was no different to sounds on that level: it's called stimulus control. With cancer detection, the smell has to produce the reaction in the dog, without any interaction from the handler.

Also, my work with gun dogs meant that I understood how they sensed scent patterns in difficult environments, following one odour among many others, just as these cancer dogs would do if properly trained.

And from training my lovely little paralysed Woody, I knew that a dog could be trained to do very complex tasks.

All these three things fed into my ideas about how to run the research. There was another element: from the very beginning I was keen to avoid contamination, and that was one of the foundation stones of the work. Everything had to be done scientifically. I don't know where this understanding came from, but I was meticulous about changing gloves after handling each sample tube of urine. Anyone helping out on this early trial, or working with me since, has to be taught to change gloves every time: we get through thousands of thin plastic gloves.

We tried to do everything correctly. We even consulted vets to establish that sniffing urine samples would in no way endanger the dogs – a laughable precaution when you think how dogs spend their days snuffling around all sorts of unpleasant smells. But we had to dot the Is and cross the Ts: we could not risk any criticism that we were in any way exploiting animals.

The original team of dogs who went into training included my puppy Tangle, a chocolate cocker spaniel with an unflappable personality, calm and hard working. He never became over-excited, was never overawed by people watching him work. He was an undemonstrative,

self-contained dog who never demanded lots of attention
or lavish praise.

I bought Tangle because I knew that, although Dill had
helped me be sure in my own mind that dogs could do this
work, he was too old to be used in a trial, and I wanted a
young spaniel to train for the work. I hadn't kept any of
Dill's puppies, except Woody. When you are surrounded
by lovely dogs, you never think about preserving their
lines, until it is too late.

I have a friend called Frances Brooks who lives up
in Scotland, and who I met when I was training gun
dogs. I was always interested in Scottish gun dogs, as
they have strong working lines there, but many of them
are trained by the old-fashioned methods I don't like.
I saw an advert for Frances and her dogs, and it said
she was using positive training methods, so I gave her a
ring. We hit it off straightaway, and she invited me up
with my dogs so that we could go out training together.
It was on my second visit that she mentioned she was
going away for a couple of weeks and had found a young
man to look after her kennels. She'd checked his refer-
ences, and she was confident he would be good. She
mentioned his name: Rob Harris. Life is full of twists
and turns and coincidences, and as you will hear later,
Rob Harris was to become an important person in
my life.

. One day, Frances rang up and asked if I wanted a puppy,
as she had a chocolate-brown boy puppy I could have.
It was exactly the right moment for me, and so I drove

up to Dumfries and Galloway to see him. Tangle was an exceptional dog: perhaps the best-behaved dog I have ever encountered. From that very first meeting, when he was tiny, he had the demeanour of an old man, as if he had been around a long time and knew the world well. Most working cockers are a bit headstrong and need training. Even though they are intelligent and quick to learn, they'll take advantage if they can get away with it.

Mr T was never like that. I barely had to train him. He trotted along beside me wherever I went, never chased anything unless he was supposed to chase – if I took him on a gun-dog shoot he'd hunt well – and I don't think I ever heard him bark. I named him after Tanglefoot beer, which is brewed in Dorset, and which was a favourite drink of mine when I was younger.

He fitted in with the other dogs in our home, but he was never a particular favourite of the others. If anything, they seemed indifferent to him. They didn't boss him about, which sometimes happens when a young puppy comes into the mix, but they didn't engage with him, nor he with them. Looking back, I think the fact that Woody needed so much attention from me, being picked up a lot, meant that Tangle simply accepted his place and trotted happily alongside me.

He took to the cancer-detection training straightaway, and throughout his life he was always very focused when he was working.

Biddy was another cocker spaniel living with me and Andy, and Andy trained her. She was smaller than Tangle, bred in Scotland as a gun dog. Another Scottish gun dog was Jade, a black Labrador.

The third spaniel was Bee, another small female cocker, but this time black. She was cheeky, naughty, extrovert and loved attention. Eliza, a seven-year-old papillon, a miniature breed, was an unusual choice. Papillons are not normally used as working dogs, but they are, in fact, toy spaniels, so we hoped Eliza would do well. She did not let us down.

Toddy was a five-year-old mongrel with a reddish coat, who at first seemed to be the most trainable and successful of our team. He worked through the samples very quickly, identifying the right one, whereas Tangle seemed to spend a few seconds on each, sniffing them carefully, before making his decision.

There were two others at the start of training: Titch, a two-year-old female Jack Russell, small even for her breed – hence her name. She had been abandoned and a rescue centre gave her to Hearing Dogs, but she wasn't suitable for the work there. I took her home and rehabilitated her, and we tried to use her for the study, but she simply didn't get it. I found a lovely family for her. There was also Reef, a German wire-haired pointer puppy, only ten months old, who was being trained for agility competitions. He dropped out because the time commitment for his busy owner was too great.

We used tea and fruit in our first scent training, using the same techniques I'd tried with Dill. We devised our own testing equipment, which we called plates. These are stainless steel dishes with plastic flowerpots clipped on top, a disposable way of making sure the sample did not move around. I spent many evenings cutting the tops off the flowerpots, which I bought in bulk from a garden centre. Soon some of the dogs were easily detecting the pots that contained oranges from those that contained other fruit, and others had mastered the Earl Grey tea test.

I was still very nervous when, in April 2002, our very first cancer samples arrived. Had we done more harm than good teaching the dogs these other smells? Would they be able to switch to the vital (but indistinguishable to us) smell of cancer? I really wasn't confident, but at the same time I had a profound sense that whatever we discovered could change the world, by proving that cancer had a recognisable smell.

We were having the weekly get-together of the cancer-detection team when the samples came. Hearing Dogs for Deaf People were, as usual, generous with their premises. We only worked outside their hours, but they gave us a suitable place to meet and, eventually, to carry out our scrupulous, monitored trial.

Carolyn came in, wearing a white lab coat and carrying a coolbox. The very sight of her, kitted out so scientifically, made me realise that this was it: from here on the trial was in earnest.

A hush fell over all of us, except the dogs. Although they are well trained, we never repress their natural curiosity and playfulness – these are attributes that make them suitable for the work we want them to do. They were not particularly impressed by a white coat, and continued to playfight and wander around the room greeting each other and all the humans, tails wagging with enough energy to power a small electricity station.

Carolyn ran through the protocols. We were to wear gloves at all times when handling the samples and were told that no pregnant women could take part in the experiment.

The samples had been frozen down to minus 35°C. They had been donated by patients with bladder cancer, some of them terminally ill, but all prepared to help a research project that could, one day in the future, help save the lives of others with the same cancer. None of us have ever lost sight of the generosity of our donors. Thirty-six patients, twenty-three men and thirteen women between the ages of forty-eight and ninety, gave urine samples. In the beginning, our control samples came from any young person who was prepared to give us one: it had to be a young person because we did not want to risk one of our controls unknowingly having cancer.

For these samples – the clear ones we would use as controls – I was given permission to recruit donors at a local sports centre, setting up a small table and handing out sample pots to young people as they walked in or out. Bladder cancer is vanishingly rare in people under forty, and these youngsters were all clearly healthy, and on the whole happy to donate samples to me after I explained what it was all about, although there were a few who were embarrassed to be asked. I carried sterile pots with me all the time, and little freezer bags to put them in.

In the very early days, most of us on the project, including me, also donated samples. It was odd because the dogs clearly recognised their owners' smells on the samples, but they mostly just gave a puzzled pause, glancing at their owner, and moved on, continuing to search out the cancer smell. Later, when the dogs were constantly finding the cancer samples among the clear, healthy controls, Carolyn also provided samples from older people who had been tested for bladder cancer and found negative, which made our work much harder, as there were plenty of other odours in there to distract them. However, it was also much more realistic: if the work we were doing was ever to be used in a practical way, the dogs would have to detect cancer from among many other odours. Commonly, but not always, patients with bladder cancer will have urinary infections and blood in their urine: we had to be certain these were not the markers that the dogs were finding. I was strangely excited when I encountered any friend, colleague or member of the family who had a urinary tract infection or who was menstruating, begging them for a sample, and confirming that I was, indeed, the mad dog lady.

Two of the dogs were trained on dried urine samples: we wanted to establish if this was an equally good way of detecting cancer.

Before we could introduce them to controls, we had to make sure the dogs were familiar with the smell of cancer.

We had weekly meetings, when samples were handed out. All four trainers took samples home, defrosted them, and got busy teaching the dogs to recognise them. The bottom drawer of my freezer always contained a few urine samples: I've never been known for my cooking skills, but all who knew me and what I was working on were even more wary about eating at our house at this time.

At first, after familiarising the dog with the smell, I concealed the sample in a plastic ball which I hid around the room, at the same time hiding other balls that did not contain a sample. Then we moved on to the plates and flowerpots: after each sample was used, the urine and the flowerpot were thrown away and the plate scrubbed.

We trained the dogs for seven months before the proper trial. John, although not himself a dog trainer, loved coming to see the dogs working. He was heavily involved in the protocols: getting ethics approval, obtaining samples, getting permission from patients. It was his dream, too, and he loved seeing the dogs demonstrating their skills.

The Big Trial, organised by Carolyn and John, took place in the late summer of 2003. It was during this training that something remarkable happened, although at the time I was very puzzled by it. Tangle loved the training. I would take him into the room where the samples were lined up, and with a 'Seek, seek, Tangle!' from me, he'd set about smelling the flowerpots, alerting me by lying down at the one that contained a positive sample. Time after time after time he got it right, outperforming all my expectations, and he was given a small treat and an extra play session as a reward.

But one day he lay down in front of the wrong sample.

'No Tangle, keep on,' I told him, hoping he would move on to the correct one. He reluctantly moved along the line and lay down in front of the positive sample, but before I could congratulate him he went back to his original choice.

I tried again, the following day, with the same sample among the others. Once again, Tangle singled it out. What's more, he was so determined to choose it that it seemed to throw him off completely; he didn't want to go down the rest of the line. He kept looking at me, as much as to say: 'What am I doing wrong?'

I stayed awake thinking about it. Why can't he do it?

Luckily, the consultant urologist who had helped us obtain samples came to see how we were getting on with the training. On the whole, I had nothing but positive feedback for him. Except for Tangle's sample.

'There's a strange problem with Tangle,' I told him. 'He keeps stopping at one of the control samples, and he's unhappy about leaving it. I've checked, and according to our records of the codes it is definitely from someone who has been cleared of having cancer.'

He took a note of the code number on the sample, and about ten days later he rang me. The patient who gave that sample had been cleared of possible bladder cancer after a cystoscopy (a camera in the bladder) and other tests had not revealed anything suspicious. But because of

Tangle's behaviour, he called him back in for further testing, and an ultrasound scan showed he had a tumour on one of his kidneys. Luckily it was at an early stage, and his kidney was successfully removed.

Incredibly, Tangle had been telling us the right thing all along: there were cancer cells in the urine, although not from bladder cancer. I felt bad that I had doubted him: I put the sample out again for him, and this time when he found it he got his usual reward. He looked at me as much as to say: 'About time. I've been telling you. You took no notice, but I was telling you . . .'

A few weeks later, a letter arrived, addressed to Tangle. 'Dear Tangle, thank you for saving my life . . .' It was from the patient. Of course, we don't know for certain that Tangle saved his life, but it's quite likely, as the other tests had been negative. If the cancer had developed, he might not have been eligible for treatment.

I shed tears when I read the letter. This was what the work was all about: actually saving lives, finding cancer that other tests missed, finding it faster than other tests, and a lot less intrusively. I can't thank Tangle enough: it was the reassurance we all needed that one day the work would have real, tangible benefits. We had no idea back then how long it would take.

This was the first time we knew that from urine we could detect more than just bladder cancer – we now know that the dogs can pick up prostate and kidney cancer as well. But for the purpose of this initial research, it was only bladder cancer that we were looking for. One step at a time.

It is easy to forget now how difficult it was, how few cancer samples we had, and how much confidence Tangle needed to stick by his assertion that we had wrongly assigned one of the samples as clear of cancer, when he could tell it wasn't.

We did dry runs of the full-scale test, tweaking aspects of the training and monitoring how the individual dogs were getting on. Toddy the mongrel seemed to be top of the class, with a very high hit rate for detecting cancer.

Finally, with ethics approval, the day of the Big Trial arrived. I was very nervous: I was sure the dogs were working well, but would it be good enough to justify further research? Had we all been wasting our time? I didn't sleep the night before, and when we set off I gave Tangle an extra cuddle and told him to do me proud. Carolyn arrived with the samples, which were all from patients new to the dogs, to eliminate any chance of them remembering a scent which they had, on a previous occasion, been presented with.

The test was done blind: we, the dog trainers, had no idea which samples were from patients with cancer, and neither did anyone else involved in the work, which by now included John's son Martin, another medic, as well as his daughter Susannah. There were 9 positive samples and 108 from other volunteers, across an age range of 18 to 85. Some of the controls were healthy, others had diseases, with blood or protein in the urine – but, crucially, they did not have bladder cancer. It was vital that the

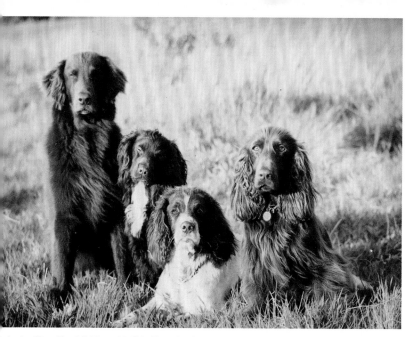

e family of four: *(from left)* Minstrel, Dill, Ruffles and Tarka.

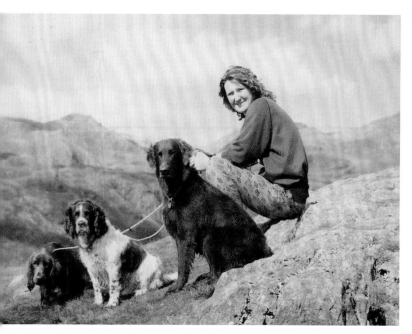

n left) Tarka, Ruffles, Minstrel and I. Tarka was very bright and worked out how to manipulate both Ruffles Minstrel.

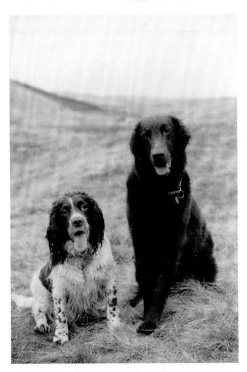

Left Good cop, bad cop: the inseparable pair, Ruffles and Minstrel.

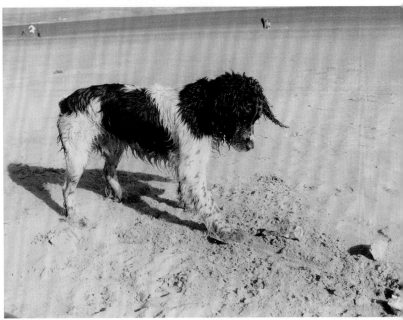

Ruffles playing his 'paper game' on the beach. He would practise his own internal control, waiting for the wind to blo the paper away while 'sitting and staying'.

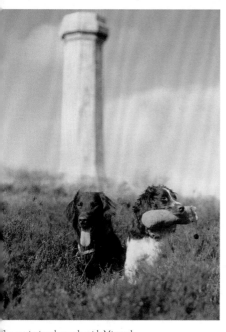

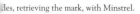
les, retrieving the mark, with Minstrel.

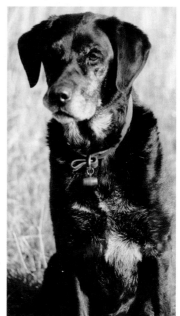

Our first family rescue dog, Liza.

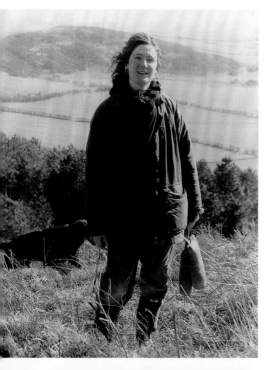

Training with the dogs at my favourite hill in Dorset.

My super dog Dill wins his first big cup. He went on to eventually win the title 'Dog Brain of Britain'.

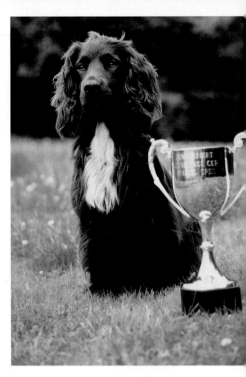

Right Dill was always keen to help out in the office! I had trained him to be a demonstration dog at Hearing Dogs. *Photograph courtesy of* Dogs Today

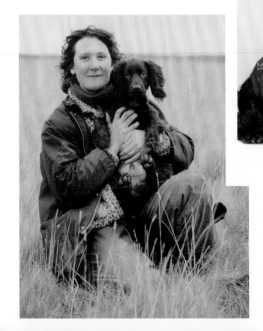

Left Dill and I, back when he was a puppy. He was a remarkable gun dog.

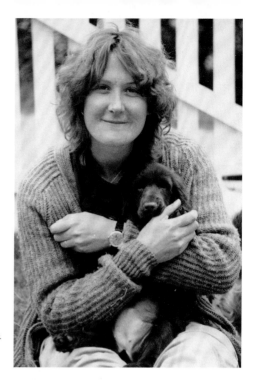

Me with Tarka as a puppy.

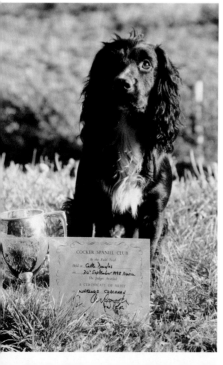

Much-loved Oak (half-brother to Dill), clicker trained with his first trial award.

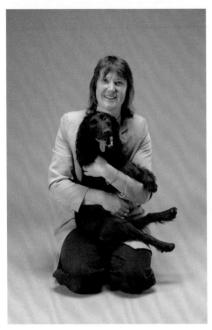

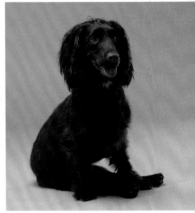

Above The most amazing, wonderful, awe-inspiring, determined little character I have ever met: Woody. *Photographs courtesy of* Dogs Today

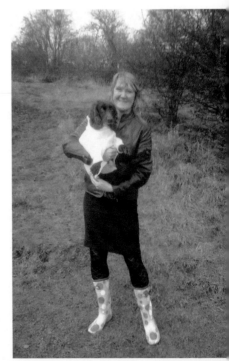

I saved Woody and Woody saved me. We had a very special relationship.

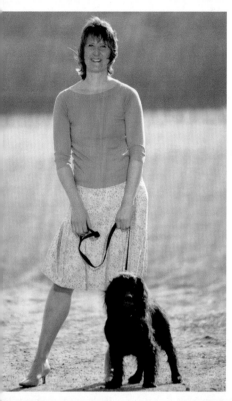

Left Tangle: the first star of the bio-
detection dogs. *Photographs courtesy of
Daily Mail/Bucks Hospital NHS Trust*

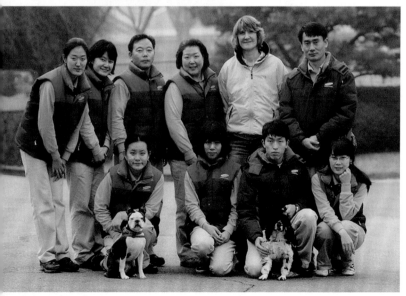

and the team at the Assistant Dogs Centre in South Korea. The work there was tough, but important.

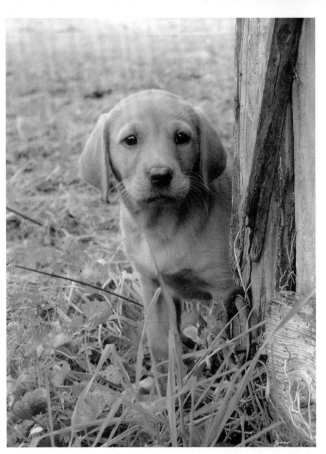

One of my very special dogs, Daisy, as a puppy. I remember the first time I saw her; she was very calm, and looked up at me and held my gaze. *Photograph courtesy of Bridget Wood*

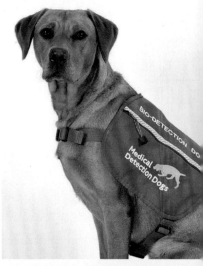

Florin, Daisy's niece. She was already working as a bio-detection dog at one year old. *Photograph courtesy of Emma Jeffery*

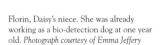

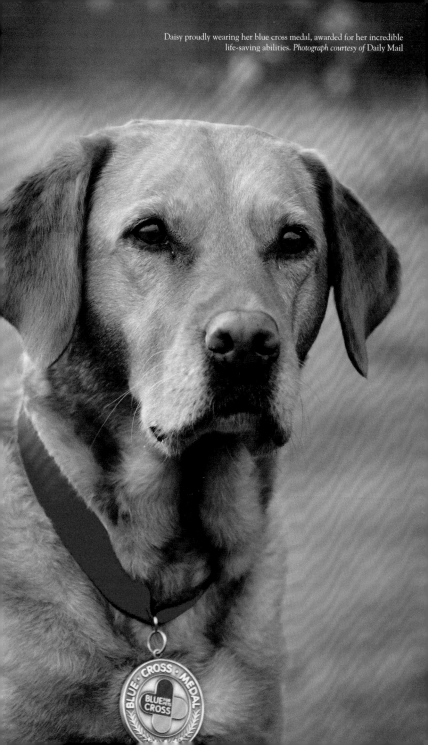

Daisy proudly wearing her blue cross medal, awarded for her incredible life-saving abilities. *Photograph courtesy of Daily Mail*

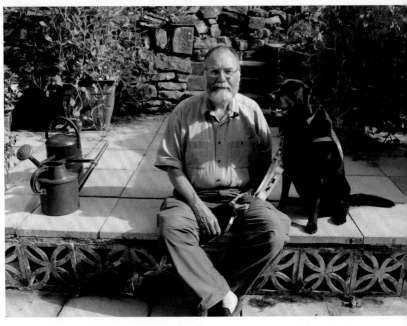

Above Some of our successful partnerships include Cherry and Zeta, our first qualified diabetes alert dog…

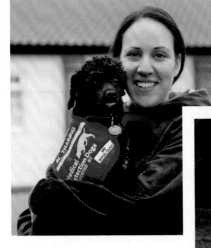

Left …Yasmine and Nano: the first nut allergy dog to be trained in Europe…

Right … and Gemma, her parents, and her dog Polo. Gemma was seven when her mum got in touch with us, and Polo has changed their lives by monitoring her blood sugar levels. *Photograph courtesy of Nigel Harper*

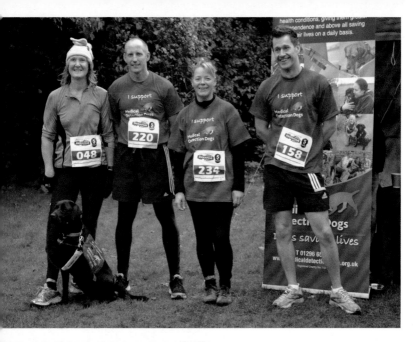

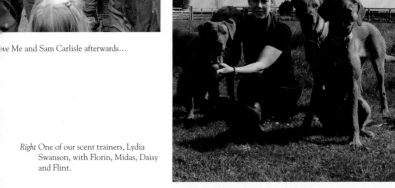

Above The Medical Detection Dogs team about to compete in the Swanbourne Endeavour. Rob Harris is to my left.

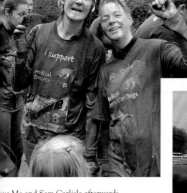

...ve Me and Sam Carlisle afterwards…

Right One of our scent trainers, Lydia Swanson, with Florin, Midas, Daisy and Flint.

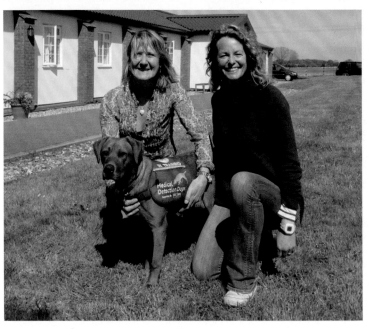

One of our lovely ambassadors, Kate Humble, with Florin and me.

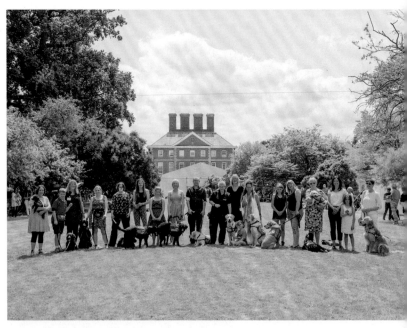

Some of our clients and volunteer puppy socialisers at the Winslow Hall summer party in 2015. I love seeing how our work has changed lives. *Photograph courtesy of Nigel Harper*

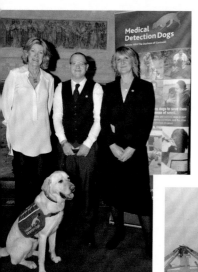

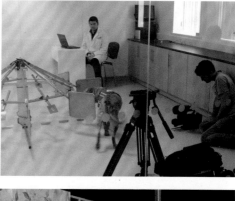

Below Channel 5 filming Daisy on the carousel. She still performs under pressure!

ve Me and Chris (with his diabetes alert dog Jade) and the Duchess of Westminster at Eton Hall. *Photograph courtesy of David Sharrock*

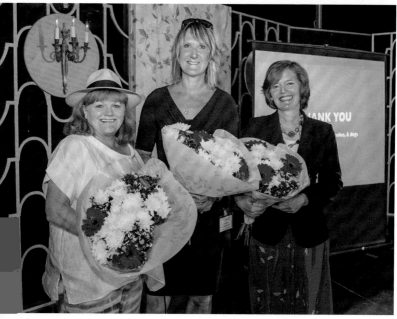

y Nicol, me and Betsy Duncan Smith at Winslow House. I am so appreciative of everything our lovely ambassadors upporters do for the charity: it has opened many doors. *Photograph courtesy of Nigel Harper*

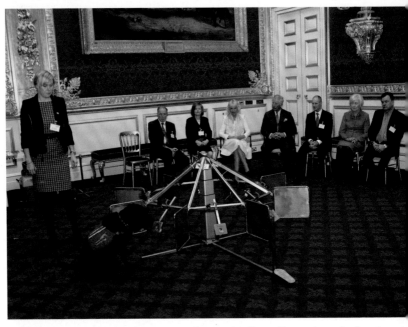

Lydia Swanson and cancer dog Lucy demonstrating on the carousel at Clarence House, with a royal audience! An amazing moment. *Photograph courtesy of Paul Burrow*

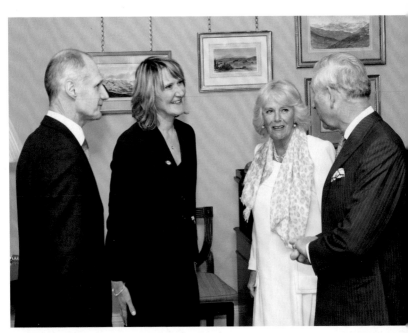

Michael Brander (chairman), me, the Duchess of Cornwall and Prince Charles, who was very impressed by the way our work is so scientifically monitored and evidence-based. *Photograph courtesy of Paul Burrow*

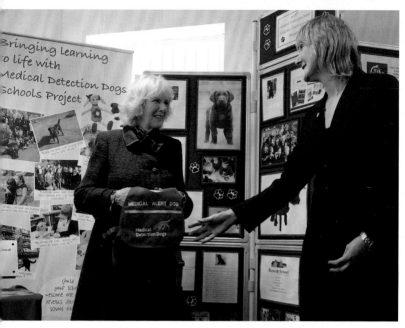

Duchess of Cornwall visiting us at Medical Detection Dogs. We only had a week to turn a derelict unit a space fit for royalty. *Photograph courtesy of Natalia Baker*

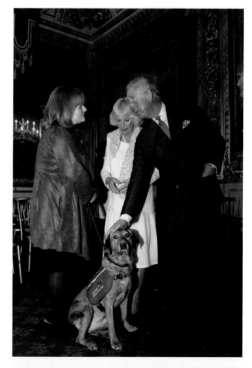

Daisy impressing Prince Charles and the Duchess of Cornwall, with Lesley Nicol. *Photograph courtesy of Paul Burrow*

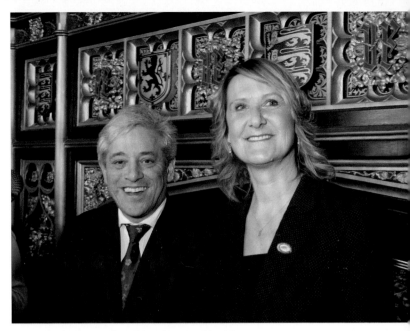

The Speaker John Bercow and me. *Photograph courtesy of Terry Moore*

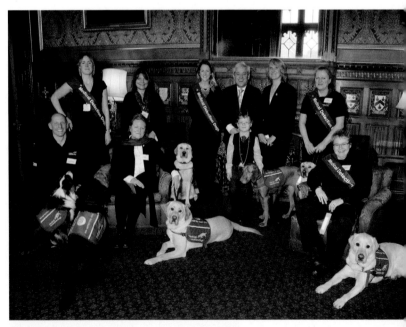

A reception at Speaker's House in 2016, which John Bercow kindly hosted. It is touching to see how moved people become when they see the dogs at work. *Photograph courtesy of Terry Moore*

dogs recognised the specific scent of cancer, not any other bladder problem.

Using our plate system, with one positive sample in a lineup of seven, the dogs approached them exactly the way we had trained them. We watched as they sniffed along the line, signalling by lying or sitting in front of the sample they thought was positive. We could not reward them, as we did in training, because we had no idea whether they were right or not, and it was clear they were puzzled by this.

There was a sigh of relief when it was over. We had no idea how well we had done, but some of the dogs had been so positive in their responses that we felt sure we had scored a higher-than-chance identification.

A statistician worked on the results to make sure everything was done correctly. We had a nail-biting few days: I found it hard to concentrate on my normal workload at Hearing Dogs. Had we cracked it? At some moments I was sure we had, at others I was totally despondent.

Finally, I got the news in a phone call from Carolyn that the code on the samples had been broken, and we had successfully proved that dogs can detect cancer at a much higher rate than chance. Chance would have meant they were right 14 per cent of the time, and as a group we had achieved 41 per cent.

I cried when I heard the news, then I gave Tangle an extra special cuddle. My good little boy had always been so willing and enthusiastic about his 'work'. The phone started ringing as the news spread among the others involved in the trial, and we indulged in the elation, savouring the feeling that we – and our dogs – had done something remarkable.

Today, working with dogs that routinely have as high as 93 per cent success rate, I look back and think the results were not so good. But there were some interesting side conclusions. The dogs who had trained on dried urine did not do as well as the others, and one dog in particular let the whole side down. His name? Toddy, the mongrel whose training had made us think he was a star. When his owner found out that of nine samples he had only correctly indicated one, she was very upset. She had worked very hard, and I was gutted for her. I have since worked out the problem: when he was being trained he was simply 'remembering' the samples for which he had previously been given a reward. In training, we had needed to use samples from the same patients, and he remembered their scent because he had a brilliant memory, rather than detecting the cancer. He was detecting the people, not the disease. Faced with completely unknown samples, he was flummoxed. Realising this helped us build even more safeguards into the training of our detection dogs.

Without Toddy, our success rate would have been much higher. Our top two dogs, Tangle and Biddy, both cocker spaniels, had a hit rate of 56 per cent each. Eliza, the papillon, did remarkably well, too, perhaps in honour of her spaniel roots, and so did Bee. Jade the Labrador was not so good, but she had trained on the dried specimens.

Looking back, there were lots of ways in which I was naïve about the design of the test, and I would do many things differently today. But we were walking through treacle in those early days.

It was a year later, in September 2004, that the official report of our experiment appeared in the *British Medical Journal*. It was a very proud day because it meant that I was no longer 'the mad dog woman', but I could show we were working on something demonstrably, scientifically worthwhile. There was a flurry of media interest and, capitalising on my experience with Dill, I'd prepared Tangle to face the cameras. I knew we would need a demo dog, so I desensitised him to cameras flashing in his face, and working under the bright lights of television cameras. I knew that if our work was going to go anywhere, we needed a massive amount of publicity. He became the face of Cancer Dogs, as it seemed as if every television station in the world wanted to film him at work. His picture was beamed around the world, and to this day the picture of Tangle with his nose down, sniffing, is the symbol of the charity on all our literature. He took it all with stoical equanimity. He was friendly with all the strangers who appeared, but he would check in by looking at me, then simply go about his business demonstrating what we were doing. I could take Tangle anywhere at any time: he never once let me down.

To my surprise, our success did not change many preconceptions. I expected, naïvely, that the scientific and medical communities would beat a path to our door, keen to provide funding and resources for us to carry on with our work. After all, more than 5,000 people die from bladder cancer in the UK every year. I thought my hand would be bitten off by every cancer hospital in the world wanting to set up centres with trained dogs. It didn't happen. After six to eight weeks of full-on media work, interest died away, and no big offers of funding came in. It was much further down the road that we gained enough support to take the work onwards on a professional footing. But we didn't give up.

CHAPTER SIX

South Korea

The little dog looked at me with his big, serious eyes. His tail was wagging so hard his whole body moved. He licked my hand appreciatively.

'I'm sorry, little chap, but I have to put you back.' I lifted him and felt his body tense as I carried him back to his cage, one of a bank of pens, four high, lining the walls of the rescue centre.

'In you go,' I said to him as he clung to me, his claws digging into my arm in a desperate refusal to go back to his captivity. 'I'm so sorry,' I said, tears pricking my eyes.

The dog was one of many hundreds I met during three visits I made to South Korea. He wasn't special: he was a lovely dog and would have made a great family pet, but he was one of many.

If you ask anyone what they know about Korea, one of the first things they say is: 'They eat dogs, don't they?'

Yes, they do. So why was I here? How could I work in a country where dogs are farmed for their meat? This is how it happened.

For two years after the trial results were published, I continued to work full time at Hearing Dogs. We carried on with the cancer research, often at home on the kitchen floor, but we also used Hearing Dogs's premises, and for a time there was even a discussion with them about our work being incorporated under their charity heading, as an offshoot of their work. In retrospect, I'm very glad this didn't happen.

I felt very flat at this time. My marriage was beginning to unravel, but I closed my eyes to what was happening because I was so desperate for it to work. I couldn't contemplate life without Andy, and I always felt I was so lucky to have him. My default position was that I could get through anything if he was by my side, and I never for a second thought I would not spend the rest of my life with him. I'd given all my emotional commitment to him.

I also faced a big dilemma: did I take the high risk of leaving Hearing Dogs in order to enable the setting up of a new charity, or not? Then maybe I'd just be known as the woman who once proved that cancer has an odour and that dogs can detect it.

Several people said to me: 'It's all very interesting, but it's not going to go anywhere, is it?'

Another variation was: 'Even if dogs can smell cancer, how on earth are you ever going to apply it?'

But I knew I could not let it go. John Church was still boundlessly enthusiastic. Mum and Dad were tremendously supportive: from the very beginning they sensed this was what I really wanted to do with my life, and they encouraged me to ignore the disappointment and to carry on with the research. They believed in what I was doing, and that made a tremendous difference to me.

In 2006, we had several meetings, discussing how to set up the organisation we initially called Cancer and Bio Detection Dogs (it later became Medical Detection Dogs, or MDD). Dad was a really important member of the team, later using his legal expertise to guide us through the tricky minefield of becoming a charity. Dad qualified as a solicitor as a young man, and then pursued a career in local government, eventually becoming the youngest ever chief executive of a local authority.

I knew that breaking with Hearing Dogs would be a great wrench but eventually I felt I had to. The cancer project was going nowhere without greater input from me and I believed the work had the ability to make a major difference to mankind.

One of the things that helped crystallise my decision was that it had become uncomfortable working there. Andy had by this time taken a senior position with another charity, but left behind a legacy of rumour and allegations that he had been unfaithful to me, which all my colleagues knew. And after a change in Hearing Dogs's administration, we were no longer able to use their premises for the cancer-detection work, which meant I no longer had that tie to them.

Another breakthrough that confirmed my decision to leave came when Bucks Healthcare NHS Trust started to talk to us about the possibility of a follow-up study funded by a grant from a charitable trust. One of the main criticisms of the first study, and a very valid one, was that we did not use specialist trained dogs. The answer to why we didn't is simple: we did not have any, only the dogs we trained in the seven months before the trial, which were of assorted breeds and backgrounds. The trust now wanted to see if we could replicate the results with a bigger sample size and dogs specially selected for their ability. They said they would need to put the new study through ethic assessment, but they would have funding from the charitable trust to pay for me to work on the project one day a week.

My decision to leave Hearing Dogs was endorsed by Andy, who had a good salary and offered to support me financially when I gave up the security of the monthly salary cheque. I still believe passionately in the work of Hearing Dogs, and after working there for nearly twenty years I feel nothing but gratitude for the opportunities they gave me, and the support we had in the early days of the cancer-detection work, but it was time to go.

Leaving gave me time to concentrate on setting up a proper framework for the cancer-detection work. We all agreed that we needed to set up a charity, but it still seemed like a pipe dream. I knew many of the pitfalls, having been at Hearing Dogs from the days when there were only four staff, but Hearing Dogs had the advantage of an American model to work from. If we set up a charity for dogs detecting cancer, we were pioneering again, in unknown territory. Dad and John were determined to make it happen, and Dad started researching everything we needed to do.

In the meantime, I carried on working with the dogs, waiting for the funding to come through. By this time, I had another dog in training, a fox-red Labrador called Daisy. Daisy is one of my soul mates: when I look back on my life, all my dogs have been very special, but I have had four soul mates: Ruffles, Dill, Woody and Daisy. Although Tangle was very, very special, he never quite occupied the same deep corner of my heart that these dogs do.

I decided to get Daisy because I knew I needed another dog to run alongside Tangle, who was two years old when I got her. I wanted a puppy to train for the discrimination work, so I needed a dog with drive. I knew it was very unlikely I'd get another cocker as calm as Dill or Tangle: cockers can be quite fizzy and distracted when they are little. The scent work requires the dog to make quite complicated decisions, and that's not possible if they are all over the place. For some reason I had a picture in my head of a fox-red Labrador – the fox reds are a strain of the standard yellow Lab, but much darker and redder in colour. They fell out of fashion for many years, and at the time they were still relatively rare, and none of the breeders I knew had any fox reds.

However, I saw an advert for a fox-red puppy, and although I'm hesitant about buying from breeders I don't know, I was reassured because the advert said the puppies were from the 'Endacott' line, which is one of my favourite lines for Labradors.

I gave the number a ring, said that I was looking for a dog to train for cancer detection. The woman I spoke to warned me that the only fox-red puppy in the litter already had a potential owner, but I was invited to see the puppies, in case the sale fell through, and because she thought I might like another puppy she had. I drove to Kent expecting to find a gun-dog breeding kennel, which I feared would be grotty and upsetting. But it was the opposite: a lovely lady called Bridget Wood had bred the puppies and they were living in her kitchen, next to the Aga. She had a gun-dog bitch who had been mated with a field-trial dog, so it was a really good litter. We took the puppies out for a walk in her quaint, rambling garden and I explained more about the work I was doing. She showed me another puppy which was available, but I told her I particularly liked the fox red, who was a very calm puppy who looked up at me and held my gaze.

'She's yours,' Bridget said.

'But I thought you said she was taken.'

'I said that so I had a get-out if I didn't think you were a suitable owner,' she said. 'You never know what people are going to be like when they ring, so I give myself a get-out clause.'

Good for her: I understood entirely why she did it. Daisy was her favourite puppy, and she had a feeling she was going to go somewhere special. I was thrilled when she said I could have her. Daisy has gone on to be the best bio-detection dog we have had, and works consistently at up to 93 per cent in training and testing. She's proved to be a gentle, placid, beautiful, loyal and amazing friend and companion. Bridget, who bred her, is a distinguished artist, who has done portraits of dogs for the Queen among many others, and a few years later she did one for me, of Daisy. It is a wonderful picture: it really captures everything about Daisy, her soul.

I still had to earn a living, so I worked on a research project for Guide Dogs for the Blind as a freelance consultant, and did canine behaviour work, getting referrals from everyone who knew me in the field. One day a week was devoted to training the cancer-detection dogs, working mainly with Tangle and Daisy. I also spent evenings and weekends on it, and I refined our training techniques, even though I was working on the floor in our kitchen, which wasn't the best place. Tangle and I were still being invited to give demos all around the country, and I was giving talks, again conquering any qualms I had about standing in front of a room full of strangers by concentrating on the work and Tangle. When I'm talking and demonstrating with a dog, it's as if I'm in a protective bubble, and my own ego, shyness and personality are completely unimportant. My passion for the work and the need to show people what dogs can do takes over, and that's all I care about.

Andy and I bought a new canalside cottage. I felt good about the move, and happier about our future than I had for some time. Buying the house was part of a new start, with both of us no longer working at Hearing Dogs and me with more time to pursue my passion. But, at the same time, I sensed that Andy's interest in the cancer-detection work was waning, which I put down to him being absorbed in the challenges of his new job.

One of the aspects of the research that intrigued me was that the dogs were showing clear interest in the samples that contained other diseases, not cancer. They sniffed these samples with a lot more interest than they took in the clear, healthy samples from young people. Because they were trained to look for cancer, they moved on to alert in front of the right sample, but we found it was much harder to train a dog to ignore samples with other illnesses in them. I realised this showed they could detect anything unusual in urine.

Surely this had to be of interest?

Again, it was John and my dad who agreed with me and encouraged me to think of other ways to work with the dogs' amazing sense of smell. Years before, Dad and I had protracted serious discussions about training pigeons to alert when intruders were in a particular secure council site. I was sure I could do it, but we never got round to trying it. Still, it showed how Dad had complete faith in my ability to train animals, and he never thought I was mad. Lots of other people did, though, and it was a struggle keeping the faith.

Before the new study started in earnest I tried out dogs to make sure I had the right ones, as this new study was to be based on using specially selected dogs. Tangle was an obvious choice, as was Daisy. I also had Oak, a relative of my beloved Dill. He was the spit of my old Oak, so I named him after him. There was another Labrador called Victor who was being rehomed. I soon realised he was not suited to the work, which showed to me that breed alone is not a sufficient indicator of how well a dog can do this specialised detection. Now I understand much more about what makes a good cancer-detection dog, so a failure like Victor was actually a valuable part of my learning process.

I trained Daisy, Tangle and Oak in the sitting room of the new canal house, which was very hard because it is a two-man job, with one person knowing which are the correct, cancerous samples and placing them in the line-up, while the trainer (me) is not aware where they are (important, so that I could not give inadvertent cues to the dogs). My sister Simone and Andy helped, but he was reluctant and seemed to have lost all interest in the cancer work.

It was in August 2007 that the inaugural meeting of what was to be our new charity was held in the dining room of Mum and Dad's house. There were ten people round the table, most of them chosen by John Church and me as potentially useful supporters. Dad chaired the meeting, and apart from John and me, the other seven were Donna Brander, chair of the Association of Pet Behaviour Counsellors; Michael Brander, Baron of Whittinghame, an estate owner and, by background, a solicitor; Professor

Daniel Mills, head of Biological Sciences at Lincoln University; Dr Roger Mugford, animal psychologist and nationally known pet behaviourist; Ron Souter, a retired bank manager; Roger Jefcoate, who volunteered to be our patron; and Jean Jefcoate, Roger's wife. Dad was appointed the secretary and his friend Ron Souter became the treasurer. It seemed like a great start, and we all left the meeting feeling uplifted.

Before the funding came through for the new study, I was approached by someone I knew from Hearing Dogs. They had been asked if they would be willing to provide a hearing-dog expert to work on a short-term consultancy contract in South Korea, travelling out three times for a month each time. They could not afford to release a member of staff, but recommended me. The job was funded by Samsung, the giant electronics company that dominates the South Korean economy. I, like most people, knew very little about South Korea, apart from the fact that dogs are on the menu there. It seemed, at first, like the last place on earth that I should go.

But then I thought about it. Samsung were spearheading a move to change attitudes to dogs in South Korea, partly because their chairman at the time was a dog lover, but more because they wanted to be accepted in the Western world, and they knew that one of the great stumbling blocks was our revulsion at their practice of eating dogs. With Samsung support and lobbying, the government had already passed a law banning the eating of dogs that were picked up from the streets: the only dog meat consumed had to be farmed under strict standards for slaughter and hygiene.

Although the idea of dog meat repulsed me, I understood that my objections were cultural: in the UK we eat lambs, cows, pigs and chickens, all sentient creatures, and across the Channel horsemeat is accepted on the dining table. We have a history of strong relationships with our dogs and cats as pets, but without that development they could easily have become another available source of protein, as they are in South Korea.

I thought about why I had become involved in gun-dog training: it was an attempt to demonstrate that dogs could be trained by my methods, without any need to brutalise them. Surely this was an extension of that? In Korea I would be training assistance dogs, but also advising in the dog shelters that deal with the strays on the streets of Seoul. It would be a chance, perhaps, to make a small difference.

Less altruistically, it offered free flights, free accommodation and very good pay. We needed money because I no longer had a salary. I reasoned that I would be able to carry on liaising with John Church and my dad about setting up the new charity by email and phone, as another bonus was that Samsung supplied unlimited free telecommunication access for me. It was also an exciting professional challenge: I was finding it hard adjusting to working on my own in my living room with three dogs instead of running a team of eighty people at Hearing Dogs.

The huge downside was leaving the dogs and, particularly, Woody, who still viewed me as his mother. Andy encouraged me to go. Mum and Dad looked after Woody devotedly, and a friend took Daisy and Tangle. I spoke to my contacts at Buckinghamshire Healthcare NHS Trust, and they were happy for a slight delay in the second study: there was no timeline on it. I was apprehensive because, apart from going to North and South America, I had never travelled outside Europe before, and I had never been away from my family for so long. But the prospect of visiting a completely different culture was appealing.

Before I committed to going I asked for a detailed breakdown of what Samsung expected. I knew they were generous employers in many ways, but that they demanded very hard work and total commitment from their staff. The Samsung representative in the UK went through everything with me, and I signed up.

When I arrived in Seoul I was picked up by Julie Lee who was assigned to me as an interpreter, and who, over the course of my three visits, became a really good friend. She was bilingual, having been educated in America. She went almost everywhere with me during my three separate visits to the country.

My immediate impression was how Westernised the airport is, and the city. But I felt like a giant, and everywhere I went people stared. At home I am tall, but there I was massive. Small children occasionally burst into tears when they saw me, and older children wanted to touch me to make sure I was real. Out in the countryside, outside Seoul, where Western visitors are less common, everyone was very curious.

While I was in South Korea I stayed in guest accommodation at the Assistance Dogs Centre, which is next to a huge amusement park called Everland, the third biggest in the world, which is owned and run by Samsung, and is close to the Samsung headquarters in Samsung Digital City. The park is run by the charitable arm of Samsung, although visitors pay to go in. Close by is the dogs' training facility, where the assistance dogs are trained, and where there is an education programme to help South Koreans understand how to care for dogs as pets. The guide-dog training programme had been established by consultants from the US and was running reasonably well, although there were some behavioural issues I sorted out. There were more serious problems with the hearing-dog training, which had also been started by US experts, and it was my job to improve it.

I soon came face to face with the dog-meat trade, as I was driven around. At crossroads, the car would pull up alongside open-backed trucks with metal grilles covering the back, packed with dogs. They all looked subdued, with their tails down. I even saw fox-red Labradors just like Daisy, which was heartbreaking. They were being transported from the farms where they were bred for meat, and were on their way for slaughter.

'Please don't look,' said the Koreans who were travelling with me.

'I need to look,' I said, even though it was incredibly painful.

Is it any different to the trucks full of cattle and sheep we regularly see on our motorways? To some Koreans the answer is no, and it is hypocritical, perhaps, for me to feel so saddened by it, but I knew it was part of my job to take forward the idea that dogs are companion animals, not agricultural produce. It has to be done in small steps, and I knew the country was not going to change overnight. If I wasn't prepared to help, could I honestly expect others to do it? My mantra while I was there was: 'If I make a difference to the life of one dog, it will eventually make a difference to many.'

The Assistance Dogs Centre looked exactly like any assistance dogs centre in the world, with the dogs kept in very well-appointed kennels. The weather was very hot and humid while I was there, which I initially found hard. I was also unnerved by the deference of the staff: everyone bows. I soon realised that I had to bow back, and how low I bowed was a sign of the status of the person to whom I was bowing. I got so used to it that when I arrived back at Heathrow a month later I was rather surprised that nobody was bowing to me.

I gave lectures on canine behaviour to the thirty or so staff at the Assistance Dogs Centre. I was initially thrown by their attitude to learning: they all had notebooks and assiduously wrote down what I said, and never asked any questions. When it came to watching them train, I asked: 'Why did you do that?'

'Because it is what you showed us with the dog you were handling.'

'But this dog did something different, so you have to adapt. You have to apply the skills needed for the individual dog. You need to try to understand the dog.'

They were used to treating dogs as fixed systems, all the same. Of course, some of the trainers there were really good, instinctively following the right methods. But most seemed to need to do everything by rote, according to a formula.

I had to challenge the way they learn. They were surprised when I asked them for questions. I'm used to discussing and arguing with trainers here, but what they wanted was a magic system laid down by me that would apply to all dogs.

I tried to teach them how to assess dogs, which is one of my passions. The guide dogs were coming in from America, but for hearing dogs and companion dogs they were using rescue dogs, and it's really important to assess at the beginning whether the dog is suitable. In nearly forty years of handling and assessing thousands of dogs I have only been bitten once, and that was when I took someone else's word about the dog, against my own judgement. I have never done that since.

I had to work much more quickly than I like to, but I used the same basic techniques I use when choosing dogs to work with here: to assess a dog I need to feel its energy. When I put my hands on a dog I get a strong sense of its nervous energy; I can tell if it is frightened, anxious, frustrated or has a high metabolic rate. So I was able to choose the dogs that would be most suitable for training.

Another part of my job was to train staff at the main rescue centre near Seoul City, which was also funded by Samsung. It was heartbreaking.

While the rush towards Western values is good because it is impacting on the dog-meat trade, and it has stopped strays being plucked off the streets for the pot, it has also had a negative impact. The Koreans are influenced by the Japanese, and at this time there was a craze in both countries for handbag dogs, miniature breeds carried around by women as accessories. Dogs were being bred for sale as handbag dogs: Maltese terriers, bichon frises, Lhasa apsos, shih-tzus. It was fashionable for their owners to dye them with harmless food dyes, and the more colours the better, so I saw them with blue bodies, pink ears, yellow tails. They lived in apartments, litter-trained like cats, and were always carried when they were outside. No wonder there were serious behaviour problems, which resulted in many of these dogs being kicked out on to the street, where they were rounded up by the dog catcher and taken to the rescue centre.

The centre kept every dog for seven days, then it was put to sleep, on a first-in first-out basis. More than 200 were killed every week. There were always between two and three thousand dogs, in small cages stacked on top of each other. There were a few aggressive dogs, but most were sad and desperate for human contact, and their desperation made me cry. The centre was hot and smelly, and there were far too many dogs for the staff to exercise them. Most of them were these little coloured dogs.

The staff were great, and the vet who met me on my first day there said: 'We do our best.'

They did: they treated every animal with respect, but it was a horrible job. At lunchtime on my first day they took me to a small shrine in the tiny garden. There were candles, and we all said a prayer for the dogs. The vet said: 'I hope you forgive me for what I do. I can't do anything else. How can we be like this? We, all who work here, feel terrible.'

It was very emotional, and I consoled him by pointing out that things are a long way from perfect in our country, with puppy farms and dogs being imported from Eastern Europe and our own trend for handbag dogs.

I longed to bring a couple of the dogs home with me. We took some back to the Assistance Dogs Centre for the hearing-dog training, and one little crossbreed with bright eyes and a curious manner failed to make the grade medically for training. The vets were very tough, and she was a bit older than the other recruits. They ordered that she go back to the rescue centre, where she would be put to sleep. I couldn't bear it, and was seriously working out how to ship her home, when she was adopted by a friend of one of the staff.

One day at the rescue centre, after I had assessed about 500 dogs (that's what I mean about working more quickly than I normally like to do), the vet said: 'We notice that you don't wear gloves.'

'No, I use my hands to sense the dog. I know if a dog doesn't want me to touch it, so I don't . . .'

'But what about rabies?'

It had never occurred to me to have a rabies jab before I flew out, and I did get scratched: never when I was handling the dogs, but when I was putting them back into their cages, when they scrabbled at my arms in a desperate effort to stop me pushing them back in, which I hated doing. It broke my heart: so many dogs, desperate for love and affection.

Luckily, there was no rabies in the shelter at that time, and I didn't worry because, if I had the jab then, it would not take until I was on my way home.

Pet ownership was becoming more popular, and people did come into the centre to choose a dog. But the staff were letting them choose on looks alone: I taught them to assess the dogs' temperaments so that they were rehomed on the basis of compatibility. It was completely alien to the staff to ask the new owners questions, like how much exercise the dog would get, what sort of home would it be living in, would there be small children, etc.

But by learning to match the new owners with the right dog, they were ensuring the rehoming would be successful and the dog would not end up back in the shelter a couple of months later.

I was homesick most of the time I was in Korea, even though everyone went out of their way to be kind and hospitable to me. But I missed my home, I missed Andy, and I missed my dogs, most of all my little Woody. I also missed the beautiful English countryside. When the day came to fly home I was very happy, and excited about the prospect of getting on with the cancer-detection work.

Little Woody Wood Chips gave me an ecstatic welcome home, and so did Daisy. Neither of them would leave my side. Woody was completely beside himself, leaping on me with his paralysed back legs flailing, screaming his high-pitched wail if anyone tried to take him away from me. Apparently, after I had gone, he accepted my absence but was very subdued for the first few days, searching for me everywhere.

My first two weeks back at home were mainly filled with writing long reports for Samsung, who wanted me to assess everything, including each member of staff. Thankfully, I had finished them when two terrible, life-shattering things happened.

The first was a report about our new cottage, which revealed the place was riddled with damp and dry rot. The cottage needed to be ripped apart while professionals sorted it out, and it would be uninhabitable for months.

The second, even more devastating event, was an announcement from Andy that our marriage was over. He told me in brutal, unequivocal terms that he wanted to move on to a new partner, and he spent hours – a whole, long night – dissecting our marriage and maintaining that he had never been happy with me. Despite the problems we had been having, I was knocked sideways. There had been plenty of clues, but I had buried my head in the sand, really believing that we were trying to make a new start with our lives together. Anything else just didn't bear thinking about. I listened to his tirade, numb and unbelieving. It was Hallowe'en, and the grimmest night of my life.

He left the next day, taking with him some clothing and a few bits and pieces, but leaving behind his books and photographs including his school photos and pictures of his grandmother. He never came back.

The final twist of the knife came with: 'And all this cancer dog stuff, it's never going to work. It's a load of complete nonsense and you know it. Get yourself a proper job.'

He had been closer than anyone to the early work we were doing, and to hear it dismissed like this was heartbreaking – but even that paled to insignificance compared to the loss of the man I thought of as a soul mate, and a life partner.

Suddenly I had no husband, no job that was paying me a regular wage, and a house that was in need of expensive remedial work. I sunk to the bottom of a deep dark pit, mentally and emotionally. I began to have debilitating panic attacks. On one occasion, two days after he left, I curled into a sobbing, shaking ball in the corner of the doctor's waiting room. My GP was brilliant, very supportive, and medication helped, but I was in the throes of a full-scale breakdown. When I went into a supermarket I had a panic attack: I was so used to shopping for two, looking at food items and wondering if Andy would like them. Shopping had always been about the two of us. Everywhere I looked in the aisles there were couples or families shopping together. An innocuous remark by a friendly shop assistant, implying that I was a married woman, tipped me over.

'I'm not married,' I said, although technically I still was. As I said it, I started to shake, and I had to abandon my basket and get out of the store. It felt like a big black hole opening up in front of me. I sat in my car in the car park for ages, until the trembling and crying abated enough for me to be able to drive.

I didn't want to eat, and after that experience I didn't want to go into a shop. Mum and Dad, Nicole and Simone fed me, pushing food in front of me and making me eat some of it. On my own, I braved the petrol station and bought cans of Heinz soup, milk and bread, my staple diet for at least a year. I saw a psychiatrist and I had a very caring community psychiatric nurse, but I can't remember too much about those first weeks. I was diagnosed with severe reactive depression and panic attacks, and I was told my condition was similar to post-traumatic stress disorder. I was put on a cocktail of drugs:

Valium for my panic attacks, two strong anti-depressants, a mood stabiliser and I can't remember what one other tablet was for.

Under stress I developed repetitive behaviours, and I rubbed one of my thumbnails so much that I wore a hole right through the nail and was scratching the flesh beneath it, which was constantly bleeding and very sore. I rocked backwards and forwards for hours, my mind replaying the marriage and tricking me into hoping Andy would come back, which was all I wanted. I would have forgiven him anything.

The dogs clustered around me in a little pack, somehow knowing that I needed all the help and support they could give me. Woody, my precious little friend, would snuggle up to me and give me a comforting lick when I was prostrate with grief. Looking after them was a routine I could not avoid, and it helped to save me.

I lived with the knowledge that Woody could die at any time, and I know I was very lucky that nothing happened to him at this terrible time, as it would have tipped me over the edge, I'm sure. He stayed well, happy, cheerful, demanding that I pay attention to him, never allowing me to wallow in self-pity. He always needed something: to be lifted upstairs, into the car, to sit on my knee.

I could not believe I could be in such pain and still wake up in the morning. Why was I alive when I was dead inside? Walking with the dogs was hard, as it seemed that I needed to make a conscious decision to take every step, but those were the first steps that led to my recovery. I was warned that I could be sectioned because there was a danger that I would do serious harm to myself. But I always knew I had to stay out of hospital, and stay alive, for Woody and Daisy. In my head I could envisage Tangle settling in a new home, but I knew Woody and Daisy would look for me if I wasn't there, and I simply couldn't bear the thought of it. Suicide seemed much the easiest option, and I couldn't think of anything nicer than never waking up because I could not see a future. But there was my family, and the dogs, so I never seriously considered it.

I still had to have contact with Andy because the house was being ripped apart and decisions had to be taken. But they were horrible, acrimonious phone calls, and I was eventually, months down the line, told by my psychiatrist and my counsellor that, for my own preservation, I should have no contact with him. That was terrible: I was so in thrall to him that I would rather have a difficult, painful conversation with him than have no contact with him at all. Looking back, I wonder how I, who had always been a strong person, could have become so pathetic.

CHAPTER SEVEN

It Can't Get Worse – Can It?

My second stint in South Korea was due to start in December, two months after Andy left me, and initially I wanted to cancel it. But the thought of Christmas at home, without Andy, was awful. I loved my family more than anything, but I could not see how I could get through it. Christmas at Mum and Dad's house is always a happy time, with lots of noise and commotion and silliness. I didn't want my dark presence dragging everyone down.

In the end, going away seemed the best thing to do, as I knew I would be working very hard and I hoped that would alleviate the pain – which, to some extent, it did. Flying out on Christmas Eve meant I avoided all the festivities of Christmas and New Year. I had to agree with my psychiatrist to keep up with my heavy dose of medication, and to tell my interpreter Julie about my problems and my treatment.

Christmas Day is not celebrated in South Korea, so instead of tucking into turkey I was sitting cross-legged on a wooden floor eating rice and beef and salad with chopsticks. Once again, I stayed at the Assistance Dogs Centre, but at weekends Julie would take me back to her family home.

She was married, and very keen to have children, but she had already had two attempts at IVF which had failed. I had read an article about the effects of stress on the body's ability to get pregnant, with conception far more likely if the woman is relaxed and happy. But IVF itself is very stressful, which clearly does not help. So I told her to get a collection of funny films and to watch them for the couple of days before her next IVF session. Months later, when I was back home, she sent me a photograph of her beautiful baby boy and wrote on the card: 'I don't think he would be here without you.'

I'll never know whether my advice really helped, but I hope it did.

Julie was a very strong woman and she couldn't understand why I was moping over a man who was not, in her assessment, worth it. She urged me to move forward, which is easier said than done. When she found I couldn't face going into a supermarket she said, 'That's ridiculous. You're coming with me.'

I genuinely felt terrible, faced with the bright lights and the aisles of food, even though I was on the other side of the world. But Julie thrust a basket into my hand and said: 'Go and pick what you are going to eat, Claire.'

She filled me with herbal potions, and drove me into the mountains to little villages where I was plied with special teas made with ingredients to make me feel better.

Although Julie herself is a Christian, and a strict Roman Catholic, she explained to me about the importance of astrological telling in South Korea, and told me that one of the best tellers, who was consulted by a number of big businesses and politicians, was currently in Seoul. She suggested I go along and see him, although she stressed he was not cheap. It was not the sort of thing I had ever done before, nor since.

My scientific, sceptical head said it was all nonsense, but I was in such despair that I was happy to do anything that anyone thought might help. I had to ring Mum to ask for the precise time of my birth down to the nearest minute, but she couldn't narrow it down as closely as that. I had no idea what to expect: I thought I would possibly be meeting a man with long grey hair, overgrown fingernails, in a room with crystal balls and eerie music. Instead, I met a very smart man dressed in a black jumper and trousers, and with a charismatic presence that I felt as soon as I walked into the room, Julie by my side.

He couldn't speak a word of English, and my Korean extended to 'hello' and 'goodbye'. Julie explained she would be my interpreter, and he nodded. With my psychology background I was fascinated by how fortune-telling works, and I knew that a lot of character reading was deduced from body language, suggestibility, verbal clues. But this man seemed to have no interest in looking at me, and he asked for no more information than the date, time and place of my birth.

He started writing and drawing diagrams, all very detailed. Occasionally he paused and sighed, and at those moments he looked at me briefly in an engaged way, then he started writing again. He never asked me any questions, and Julie and I sat there for twenty minutes or so, in silence.

He then announced that he was ready. He said that every life goes in seven-year cycles, and that he could tell me about my past or my future. I wanted him to tell me about my future: I was desperate to be told that Andy would come back to me, admitting he'd made a great mistake, that our separation was a blip. But I decided to ask about my past because that would be a test: I would know whether or not he got it right.

'That is easy,' he said. 'But first, can I say something? I will tell you about your past, your present and your choices for the future, but I must say to you that this is an unusual chart.'

'Why?' Julie asked.

'Two reasons. The first is what the chart is showing me, and the second is the amount of pain you are currently experiencing.'

I thought this was interesting, but didn't suspend my scepticism: perhaps my hunched shoulders were telling him that I was unhappy and hurting. He carried on: 'I'm sorry you lost your home, your job and your soul mate, but all these things had to go. They were trapping you, and you need to move to the next stage of your life. Before I tell you about the past, I have to tell you that I understand the pain. I don't often see this amount of pain at one time, normally it is spread between the zones. You have had a lifetime's pain in two or three months.'

I didn't give him any feedback: he wasn't asking for any, and he only occasionally looked at me, addressing himself to Julie more than to me. Then he embarked on my past: 'The timing of your birth was wrong, you came before your time.'

Julie said, 'What do you mean, was she born early?'

'No, no, no. I don't mean born before your time on the calendar, I mean born in the wrong time. It wasn't a good time for your parents, it caused them a huge amount of stress. You made your mother unwell during the pregnancy, she was very thin and sick, and very unwell after your birth. '

I had always known Mum and Dad were taken by surprise when she became pregnant soon after they married, and that they had no money at all, and would have preferred to wait a couple of years until Dad was qualified and working. I was surprised that he had picked up on this, and it surprised me more how accurate he was.

'You had a happy childhood but with lots of change, and this makes you cling to things you feel at home with. You have anxiety about change, and yet you have had lots of change.'

Again, he was right: I had moved school several times as my father's career progressed.

'You found a soul mate and you were happy but you have loved more than you have been loved.'

This really struck me. Andy was the one who constantly said 'I love you', and was always effusive with cards and flowers, leaving loving little notes on my pillow. I'm not by nature romantic: I have to remind myself to do romantic things. Andy was always telling me how important I was to his life, that I was the best thing that ever happened to him. But this man was saying I loved more than I was loved. I was so shocked by this that I asked for him to repeat it.

I believed I had messed the marriage up, that if I had in some way treated him better, shown more affection, loved him more, he would still be with me – this is what he told me the night he announced that he was leaving. But now I was hearing something different.

'It is true, you loved more than you were loved. But anyway, that relationship was not right for you.'

He said it in almost an offhand way.

'I will move on to the next part. I will tell you about your last two seven-year segments. You are a jewel. I don't see many jewels. For the last fourteen years you have been buried in sand, and all the grit and dust has stuck to the jewel, so the jewel cannot move forward. The only way the jewel can shine is by washing it, and the pain you are experiencing is the washing.

'When you come out of the washing you will shine, you will do what you are intended to do on this earth. But until you do, you cannot fulfil your destiny.

'Your husband was the sand and he was clinging to the jewel, and while he was clinging there was no way you would do what you are about to do.'

I was upset by this and said to Julie: 'Please tell him that I was very happily married, that I loved my husband.'

He simply repeated: 'You were in sand. What's happening now has to happen. When the jewel starts to shine, your destiny will be achieved.'

I was worried by now. He had been accurate about my childhood, but I did not care about being a jewel, I just wanted Andy back. I asked him to tell me about my future. He replied that it was hard to give details because much of it would come down to choice, but I had the potential to make an impact on mankind.

'Jewels are usually involved in saving lives, but not always. Sometimes they are people who are put here to make a change in the direction in which mankind is going.

'I don't know what you are involved in, but it is the right thing to do. It will make a difference to people all over the world and it will save lives all over the world.

'Your destiny is to do this. Forget all about your husband: your path is to do this thing, but you may resist, and I think you will because of your resistance to change. I am sad about this: you will do it in the end but if you get dragged down in the sand and dirt you will slow the process by many years. You are going to be hit by seven more sticks in the next seven years, and each stick may hurt but will get you nearer to where you should be.'

He was very animated when he talked about the jewel, losing his calm front and talking volubly to Julie, who had to keep telling him to stop so that she could translate for me. He seemed to find it frustrating and slightly annoying that he had to keep breaking his flow.

I said: 'Why can't I do this with my husband? Why can't I be back with him?'

He shrugged. 'Because that's what has to happen.'

I knew he was talking about the charity. I was emailing Dad on a nightly basis as we were deciding our objectives in terms of research and assistance dogs, and Dad was making sure we jumped through the right hoops to get charitable status. But at that time I had no idea that I would ever be able to train dogs to detect cancer on a large scale, or that we would ever get the charity up and running, or that the work would make an impact.

The teller said: 'Whatever it is, it will succeed and you must have faith and persuade others it will succeed. You will become known around the world, you will travel around the world to talk about this thing. It won't just affect your country. At first you will feel as if you are swimming against the tide, but if you go in the right direction the water will help you.'

I persisted that I didn't care about my work – all I wanted to know about was my personal life, and whether my husband would ever come back to me.

'If you want him back, it could possibly happen. I can see a man, younger than you, and he's not at all what you would expect, and he's not what you are looking for or what you think you want. You will turn him away several times. I would advise you not to turn him away because life will be much easier if you don't.'

Soon after the session was over, I rang Mum and Dad and told them all about it. I also told a friend, Peter Gorbing, the chief executive of Dogs for the Disabled, and a very down-to-earth, sensible person. He said: 'Wow! That sounds as if it's going to happen. You'd better do it then, hadn't you?'

'It's probably just mumbo jumbo,' I said.

'It sounds a bit detailed for mumbo jumbo.'

I'm very glad I did tell other people about it, because otherwise I might have wondered if I'd made it up or embellished it over time. But Peter, Mum and Dad heard straightaway, and Julie was also a witness. My scepticism has not completely abated, but I do believe this man in some way tuned in to me, and the reading he gave me applied very closely to me.

Sometimes I wish I could fly back to South Korea and have another consultation with him. But I know he would say I don't need to, because once you know your destiny (which he was clear was my work) then you will make decisions that help you towards that goal. I'm not a convert to fortune-telling: this is the only time in my life I have done anything like this, and I have never felt tempted to have my fortune told by anyone else.

It was on this visit to South Korea that I began to be interested in Buddhism, and the concept of living in the moment, an interest that was reinforced when I was back in the UK and did a course of cognitive behavioural therapy, which taught me mindfulness. It played in to my thinking about dogs, and the disputed question of whether they have insight. I became increasingly interested in something that is now talked about a lot by animal behaviourists: the fact that internal frustration is consuming, for humans and dogs, and it leads to irrational behaviour.

Dogs live in the moment more than we do, they don't ruminate about the way things were or the way they could be, which is something we human beings could learn from. They don't worry about what will happen tomorrow.

One of the dog trainers in South Korea took me out for the afternoon a few times, and we would visit Buddhist temples. By the time I made my third and final visit, I was doing the CBT course back at home, and my counsellor was very keen that I should make time to meditate while I was away. We went to a massive Buddhist temple, with a huge gold Buddha outside, and I sat there and meditated, as people came in and sat around me. There is research that shows that when you are around other people who are meditating, their energy helps to make you calm and relaxed.

I had lots of time to read while I was away in South Korea, and I read widely about dogs, and about human psychology. I took a pile of books, but also researched online. I was particularly interested in how conscious behaviours are influenced by subconscious imperatives, an area where there is a complete crossover between humans and dogs.

By the time I left Korea for good I was fond of the country and fond of many of the trainers, but it was clear there was a huge way to go in terms of changing perceptions about dogs. I can only hope I helped a bit, but I don't delude myself that I made much difference. The fashion for handbag dogs is just as disrespectful as eating them; it's the opposite side of the same coin.

I was last there in 2008, and perhaps there have been improvements since then. However, the Hearing Dogs project is closed down: although it was working, it was not embraced by the deaf community there. Interestingly, there are other countries where it does not work, mainly because they are countries where, culturally, dogs are not part of normal family life. On the whole, in the UK, we respect dogs, but where the tradition is that the dog is slave to the man, accepting the help of a dog is not easily done.

We are very privileged here: we are forward-looking about dogs. It's strange, therefore, that it has taken such a long battle to get the idea of dogs sniffing cancer accepted. Other countries are more open to it than we are.

For a few months, once I was back in the UK, everything seemed to go wrong for me, from my health to the work on the house. It was a very bleak time, and I was convinced there was a jinx on me. One of the worst incidents came when I was sitting on the canal bank outside the cottage on a sunny evening, feeding the ducks that I'd raised on the canal since they were babies. One duck, a big fat white Aylesbury duckling, was very tame, and happy for me to stroke her. I waved and shouted a greeting to the guy who lived on the canal boat moored opposite the cottage: he had become a friend, and always kept an eye on the place for me.

I was expecting a workman to fix my boiler, and I saw a van approaching, driving far too fast down the towpath. I went inside, and then heard a shout from my friend from the canal boat. The van had hit one of my ducks, deliberately he thought. I went outside and my lovely Aylesbury duck was dying, with tyre marks across her body. She was in pain, and I could see she would not survive. Knowing how to kill a duck, I wrung her neck.

As I did it, the floodgates opened, and I began to sob. But my grief was interrupted by an angry shout from a man on a boat that was going past: 'You f****** bitch, you just murdered that duck! I'm going to report you to the RSPCA.'

The man from the boat opposite leaped to my defence. 'No she did not.'

The first man was screaming obscenities, then the boiler man came out. My defender from the opposite bank gave him a mouthful, accusing him of being the murderer. He didn't try to deny it when I showed him the tyre marks on her neck.

'I'm sorry,' he said, 'I thought she would get out of the way. I was in a bad mood.'

Now the man on the boat turned his anger on the boiler man, and there was another horrible altercation.

I sat down with my head in my hands, thinking: 'I cannot go on like this.'

I remembered my grandmother telling me when I was little and very shy that I had a guardian angel who would always care for me, and that the world was not a frightening place. I said out loud: 'If you are there, angel, help me. I am not going to survive on my own. Let me know you are there.'

Eventually I recovered enough to take Daisy, Woody and Tangle for their normal walk along the towpath. As we walked along, a ray of sunshine penetrated the leaves on the overhanging trees, and in the bright pool of light I saw a tiny white feather, spinning as it descended to the ground. I picked it up, remembering being told by a friend that finding a white feather symbolises that you are on the right track in life. I held it out to Daisy, who looked at it and sniffed it softly.

Holding it carefully, we carried on with the walk, and before I got back to the cottage I found three more white feathers. Cynics can dismiss it – I was on a towpath and there were ducks living nearby – but for me the feathers really meant something. I had a feeling, for the first time, that things would get better. The house was a long way from finished, but I felt my spirits lifting slightly, and the work no longer seemed insuperable, even though I had no idea how I would be able to get it done.

My home was a building site, as the floors and skirting boards had been ripped out. The furniture was all piled up at one end. I worked on it whenever I could, but I needed help lifting things. My friend Gill Lacey, who had helped me so much in the past, was amazing. She provided a listening ear, even when I wanted to sob down the phone in the middle of the night. She must have been so bored, and so must all my friends and family, hearing me going on and on and on about Andy. Gill was also very hands-on, turning up at the cottage with rubber gloves and a bucket, and saying: 'Right Claire, we're going to get this place cleaned.'

Another friend who listened to me howling down the phone at all hours, day and night, was Pauline Appleby. I met Pauline because she was secretary to the Association of Pet Behaviour Counsellors when I was chairman, and we always worked together well. She was a good friend, but we were not especially close before. However, when I needed friends she was completely there for me. I must have tried her patience, but she never showed it, never complaining about me disturbing her sleep.

Things started to change, very slowly. My family and my good friends were so supportive, even though I put them through a lot. I'd have loved a magic pill to make me feel better, but there is no miracle cure.

One counsellor told me to think only of the immediate hour, not even a day. The idea of a whole day was too much: I couldn't bear the idea that I would still wake up tomorrow, when all I wanted was to not be there. You get to a point with depression when you realise there are only two solutions: kill yourself, or start the long, slow process of getting better. By setting targets for the hour – simple things like walking the dogs or washing my hair – I began to cope. Meditation and exercise both helped. Most of all, the unquestioning love and devotion of my three dogs carried me through. One of the best prescriptions for depression is fresh air and exercise, and because of my constant waggy-tailed companions I was forced to get out, even when I would have preferred to bury myself under the duvet.

Each day, by the tiniest increments, I became more balanced, happier, confident and motivated to carry on my work on cancer detection with the dogs. It took a long time to be completely well again, but I was finally on the road to recovery.

CHAPTER EIGHT

Healing Begins

'I think I've done it, I'm pretty sure I've trained dogs to find cancer, but I want you to have a look.'

Rob Harris was a dog trainer I respected greatly. I'd first heard his name from my friend Frances in Scotland, then I had met him when he joined Hearing Dogs as a puppy-socialising manager, seven years earlier. When Rob left school he trained as a mechanic, but he always loved dogs, and eventually took the plunge and found himself a job in an animal rescue centre, at half the salary he earned before. He then did a couple of other jobs with dogs before coming to Hearing Dogs.

I immediately recognised he was a natural, instinctive dog handler. We had a connection: Frances, who bred Tangle, was a great friend of Rob's and had given him Mungo, a Labrador he trained to work as a gun dog. We bonded over our interest in gun-dog training, and he was impressed that I was training the same dogs to be both assistance dogs and gun dogs, flying in the face of a great deal of received wisdom.

After a couple of years, Rob left Hearing Dogs to work as a handler and trainer of explosives and drugs dogs, screening aircraft cargo. Rob heard I was considering setting up a charity to detect cancer. He was fascinated by the idea, rang me up, and I invited him to come along on a Saturday and see what I was doing. I valued his opinion, especially as he was working with sniffer dogs.

'Yes, I reckon you've done it. They're finding it,' he said, as he watched Tangle, Daisy and Oak sniff out the samples in Mum and Dad's kitchen.

Rob was very keen to help, especially as his father had recently been diagnosed with prostate cancer. He took a great chance, coming on board to work with me one day a week, which later increased to two days. His bosses at the cargo-screening company were very interested in what we were doing, and were generous in allowing him to cut his time with them to three days. But they also told him he would be back. 'These projects only last a year,' one of them predicted. As Rob says: 'He didn't know Claire!'

But it was a risk for Rob: we were still at the stage where everything could have gone belly up, and we were fighting for funding.

In fact, funding was my main preoccupation at this stage, alongside the battle to become a registered charity. Our original name was Cancer and Bio Detection Dogs, which at the time we all agreed summed up what we were doing, and we were incorporated as a company in the autumn of 2007, just when my life and emotional security were going into freefall. But meeting the exacting standards of the Charity Commission was a different matter, and there were some desperately dark times when we despaired of it happening.

We were told our application had numerous technical problems, and we were unsure we could overcome them. We'd been consulting an expert on charity formation, but he could see that we faced an uphill struggle, and he didn't feel he could give the time to it that was needed. Nobody else volunteered, so it fell to Dad to take on a huge burden of work. He was reluctant, mainly because he and I are so closely related and both have prominent positions with Cancer and Bio Detection Dogs, which he feared would prejudice the Charity Commission against us. But he believed, almost as passionately as I did, in what we were doing. Mum had recently been diagnosed with lung cancer and, thank God, came through the gruelling treatment, but cancer, and especially early detection of it, was very much in the minds of everyone in the family.

Dad's background as a lawyer, and his meticulous approach to the work, was what eventually saw us through. I am so grateful for the many hours he put in for the charity. For a time it seemed that the solution was to amalgamate with another charity, but I'm so glad we didn't go down that route. Dad relied on Michael Brander, who also has a legal background, John Church and all the trustees to provide him with the fullest facts, opinions and history, and he bombarded me with questions online while I was away in South Korea. He worked very long and very hard, and eventually, in June 2008, we achieved charitable status.

Before that, John Church, Carolyn Willis from the Bucks Healthcare NHS Trust, and I made a trip to Norway to see a system being used there, training search dogs by using a carousel. This was the bit of their work we were interested in: bending down all the time to put samples on the floor was backbreaking, and we knew that if we were ever going to do research on a big scale we needed a better system of training. The carousel means the samples are off the ground, at the right level for a standing dog to sniff, and very much easier for the trainer. We came up with our own design, and were introduced by our then patron to a company that manufactures specialist equipment for people with disabilities, who agreed to make it for us. We paid for it with a generous grant from his trust fund. It is made of surgical-grade stainless steel, so we can keep it sterile.

Even more importantly, we needed premises. Working in Mum's kitchen couldn't go on, and I was still in the throes of having my house renovated. Even without its problems, that wasn't a satisfactory place to train, either. John Church gave us a generous donation, and we used some of the money from the grant for the new study, which we were doing with Bucks NHS Trust to see if we could replicate the results of the first study with a bigger sample size and dogs selected for their abilities. Carolyn

Willis, John Church and I drove around looking at different options, and eventually settled on an old MoD building on Westcott airfield in Buckinghamshire. Westcott was an RAF base during the war, and was then used by the MoD for rocket propulsion research, and is now a business park.

It had a lot to recommend it, perhaps most of all the fact that it was cheap. The company running the park was also very relaxed about having dogs around the place. The downside was that it was a single brick thick, and had a leaking roof that constantly needed patching. When it was built during the war, the drainpipes had been run inside the building for some unknown reason, and the place was fiercely cold throughout the bad winter of 2008/09, when we all wore more clothes at work than we did outside. Rob Harris checked the temperature one very cold day: it was below freezing outside but an even bigger minus number inside.

The front door was two bits of timber nailed together and secured with a mortice lock, and our funds were so precarious that we monitored the electricity meter to see if we could afford to have any heating on. I said to the others: 'If we put the heating on, I may not be able to pay you at the end of the week.'

One day I told Rob and Simone, who was working with us by then, that I only had enough money to pay them for the next two weeks, and all three of us decided that we wouldn't take any wages until there was some more money in the bank. I will never forget their commitment at this time, when the whole future of the charity was so precarious.

Because the building was originally an officers' mess, the kitchen was disproportionately large, taking up a third of the space, but this was good as we had lots of space for freezers to store our samples – though it was so cold in the winter months, we probably didn't need the freezers. The toilet doubled as a storage room, and we had to fight through boxes of equipment every time we went to the loo. We were so poor that in our first Christmas there, Dad handmade our Christmas cards and printed them on his printer.

We trained four dogs for the new study: Tangle, Daisy, Oak and one of Rob's dogs, a springer spaniel called Jake. Rob and his wife had six dogs of their own when he started work with us, which they trained for agility and field work. Jake had been assessed as a hearing dog, but rejected because he had behaviour problems, including aggression. Rob's wife Becky adopted him, rather than let him go to a dog rescue centre where his aggression would make him difficult to rehome.

Rob and Becky did a wonderful job turning him round, and he revealed himself to have a tremendous drive for search work, and under Rob became a good cancer-detection dog.

We worked on until the middle of 2010. Again, we had to wait for samples to be available. We trained the dogs four times a week, with me handling Daisy and Tangle, and Rob working with Jake and Oak. When the final test came the dogs were double-blind tested (which means we didn't know where the cancer samples were on the carousel), all the control samples were fresh, and the dogs had never encountered them before. As in the first study, the dogs were asked to find positive cancer samples among seven urine samples. The dogs were allowed a repeat run if I or Rob felt they were confused. The control samples contained other odours, caused by the donors being smokers, having blood in the urine or infections.

The results were much better than the first study, with the best dog, Daisy, correctly identifying 73 per cent of the cancer samples, and the worst dog at 57 per cent, making an average across the group of 64 per cent. As for correctly ignoring the other samples, the best dog, Oak, achieved 92 per cent success, down to 56 per cent for the worst dog. Daisy was the best dog overall, and was fast becoming our most reliable bio-detection dog, taking over from the ageing Tangle as the star of our team.

The results of this second study were later published, in 2011, in *Cancer Biomarkers*, a journal that publishes original research on the subject of identification of markers associated with cancer.

Again, what concerned us was that the performance of the dogs dropped as they did more and more runs to detect the cancer samples, simply because Rob and I were unable to congratulate them when they got it right. The scientists we were working with quite rightly did not believe the dogs should be rewarded, but dogs are not scientific instruments, and we had trained them by giving them a treat or a special bit of play whenever they made a correct identification of cancer. Now, under examination conditions, we could not give them this feedback, as we did not know ourselves whether they were right or wrong. Puzzled by the lack of interest we were forced to show, they became less enthusiastic and their success rate declined. It's fine not to reward a dog two or three times; its enthusiasm for the work remains high especially if it then gets a big reward at the end. We use this technique to increase the trained response. But after a month of working with no feedback, they clearly began to wonder what they were doing wrong, and stopped working at maximum ability.

I could see we were not getting the best out of them, but there was nothing I could do about it. It is hard to explain to people who do not own dogs that they are not standard pieces of equipment, they are biological systems that evolve by learning, and get better and better through a process of understanding what they are doing. But whenever I raised the question of rewarding the dogs I was accused of not being scientific, and being 'wishy-washy' in my attitude to research.

We felt demoralised at the end of the testing, but we had showed an improvement on our previous results. It was a frustrating time – we did not seem to be moving forward as quickly as we had hoped. In retrospect, it was a good learning curve because we realised the level of scrutiny we would be subjected to, and that has been our benchmark ever since.

Thankfully, today, with the help of a wonderful medical statistician, Steve Morant, who took on board the major failing in the testing process and devised a computer software programme for us, we can now do double-blind testing and, almost instantaneously, unlock the codes on the samples to tell us whether or not the dog got it right. The information about which samples are positive can be inputted off site, without the trainers having any involvement, so it is rigorously scientific. When the dog identifies a sample the trainer presses the number into the computer, and is told immediately if the dog has been successful, and can have a reward. This means that, even under test conditions, we now regularly score over 90 per cent correct identifications.

There are some wonderfully lucky moments in the story of Medical Detection Dogs, and one came when a young man, Richard Hartley-Parkinson, came to write about us for the *Bucks Herald*, our local paper. We had officially registered the charity by this time, but we were still in the throes of setting everything up. He listened to me explaining what we were doing, and he watched the dogs working. Like everyone who sees it, he was very impressed. He said he would write about us, and asked if there was anything we needed.

'Yes, a viewing gallery. I want to invite people in to see the dogs working, but if they are inside the same room as the dogs it compromises our results. I'd like a proper screen they can stay behind. Showing what we do is the only way we will raise funds.'

Richard saw me on one of the days when I was at my lowest ebb. My fingers were bleeding because I had rubbed right through the nail, and he came with me to buy plasters. Two good things happened. The appeal he put in the newspaper for a viewing gallery and a partition wall brought a fantastic response from a chap who simply turned up and said, 'Tell me exactly what you want, give me a week, and you'll have it.'

One of his family had died from cancer, and he generously gave his time and donated all the materials. Having a viewing gallery meant we could start running regular open days – although we always had to pray for dry weather when we invited people in, because of the embarrassingly leaky roof. The second amazing thing was that when Richard told his landlady, Sarah Boyer, about this mad dog woman he had met who was doing important work finding cancer, she realised that she knew me. She was an old friend who I had lost touch with, and she's now back in my life as a friend and a supporter of the charity.

We worked exclusively on the cancer research until early in 2008, when our work took us in an unexpected but hugely rewarding direction, more or less by chance.

I was contacted by Angela Kearton, the wife of Cherry Kearton, a reader in pure mathematics at the University of Durham. Cherry had been an insulin-dependent Type 1 diabetic since he was twenty-nine, and for many years he managed his condition very well. But as he grew older, he began to lose his awareness of when his blood sugars were out of kilter, going either too high or too low. He had a few collapses, and Angela was very worried about him whenever he went to work or to their allotment on his own. He collapsed when he was shopping, and when he was giving a lecture. He was taking Warfarin for another condition, so falls were especially dangerous to him, as Warfarin is an anti-coagulant and bleeding can be difficult to stop.

Angela feared he would have to give up his job, and that his whole life would be curtailed. She searched the internet for help, and discovered that in Australia and North America there were pioneer studies into the use of dogs to alert diabetics to blood sugar imbalances. Angela and Cherry had a lovely black Labrador, Zeta, and Angela wondered if there was anyone in Britain who would be able to train her to alert Cherry to his hypoglycaemic attacks. She began an exhaustive ring-around of dog charities, drawing a blank, until someone suggested she contact me as I might be interested.

I was *very* interested. I had noticed the cancer dogs were fascinated by other odours in the urine samples, not just cancer, even though they ultimately honed in on the cancer odour. I knew dogs could smell disease, I also knew that dogs are very happy to help their owners in all possible ways: it's a symbiotic relationship. So I could see no reason why I couldn't train a dog to alert to diabetic problems, although I'd never done it before.

It was Valentine's Day in 2008 when I made the five-hour drive to Durham, and I still thought I was going to die from grief at the death of my marriage. But work saved me: I had a project, and I moved in with Cherry and Angela for a few days. Zeta had originally been chosen to be a guide dog, and Angela had puppy-walked her for the charity, but she had failed on a minor medical ground, and they kept her as a pet. This was reassuring, as it meant that she was the right kind of dog with the right kind of basic training.

I observed her for the first day, watching her when Cherry was doing a test to check his blood sugar levels. She went quiet, and looked at him attentively. I told Cherry that every time she looked at him while he was checking his blood levels, he must praise her, and if the blood sugar was below a certain marker, he had to click the clicker and give her a treat. Neither Cherry nor Angela believed this would work, but Zeta caught on very quickly.

Angela says that the first time Zeta alerted properly, nudging Cherry without seeing him doing a test, she burst into tears. Zeta was alerting before I left after three or four days, and within a fortnight she was consistently alerting. At first, Cherry and Angela thought Zeta was making errors, until they realised that she was not only alerting to high and low sugar levels but also rapid drops in Cherry's sugar levels.

Within a couple of months, Zeta was reliably alerting even in public places, with lots of other smells and distractions.

Cherry is now retired, but when he was still lecturing Zeta became a very popular figure on the university campus. She wore one of our Medical Alert Dogs coats, which meant lots of people stopped to talk to her and the Keartons about her work – something that happens to all our alert-dog clients.

Zeta was our pioneer, the dog that launched the other half of the charity. Sadly, she has now died, but Cherry has another assistance dog living with him. We now do two things: training dogs to scientifically detect cancer, and possibly other diseases from samples; and also training dogs to live with people with diabetes and other medical problems.

As soon as I knew it was possible, after the success with Zeta, I checked out how we could do the work properly. When the story of Zeta and Cherry was covered in magazines and newspapers, I was approached by many people who either had diabetes themselves or were living with someone with the disease, and who were desperate for help. The majority of our trustees were in favour of the diabetes project but some were against it because they felt it would detract from the cancer-detection work. I felt strongly that they went together well, primarily because they both rely on olfaction, the dogs' ability to smell.

I was also keen to do something that was immediately beneficial, with a straightforward payoff. I knew from the response to Zeta's story that there was a need for many dogs to be trained to help people with diabetes, and, tactically, I felt that training assistance dogs could help support our other work. I also knew that I could get it up and running comparatively easily.

The cancer work was in its research stage and there was no guarantee that it would ever be taken up. The medical profession was still very resistant, and generally ignored our invitations to come and see what we were doing. There was a very real worry that it would all fall flat, especially after a bad day working with contaminated samples, when even I questioned what we were doing.

With the diabetes work, we could start helping people more or less straightaway, just as soon as we had time to train the dogs. The science behind the work was very much the same as the science underpinning the cancer research: metabolic changes in the body give off an odour, which the dogs detect. In the case of cancer, volatile organic compounds from the tumour are released into the bloodstream and are then excreted into the urine. With diabetes it is more straightforward: the signal of altered sugar levels in the blood is exhaled in breath. Essentially, the dog is doing the same job: finding a smell that we want to know about.

Surprisingly, there was still some resistance from the medical profession to the diabetes work, despite the models provided by other charities working with people with disabilities. But the opposition was nowhere near as entrenched as it was with the cancer work.

I contacted Assistance Dogs International, and found out what we would have to do to become an accredited member. ADI was set in 1987 to supervise assistance-dog charities, making sure the dogs are treated humanely, the clients are treated with respect and dignity and that training is professional at all times. They inspect organisations like ours for cleanliness, hygiene, our administrative procedures and how we screen both the dogs to train and the clients to place them with.

We did not qualify for immediate accreditation: we had to have successfully placed a minimum of three assistance dogs with clients. So we were in a no-man's land, but in the meantime, before we had our three dog/client partnerships in place, we chose the distinctive red coats that both our assistance dogs and our bio-detection dogs wear to this day. I knew I wanted the coat to be red. I can't explain why: I don't like red and I would never wear it myself, but it instinctively felt right. We also chose the logo of a dog sniffing, which is one of the many photos taken of Tangle, working his way along a line of samples to find the one with cancer, when the results of the first trial were published. Tangle, with his nose down, will live on forever at the top of all our literature and on the backs of all our trained dogs, a fitting memorial to him.

Now I had to find dogs to train to be assistance dogs. I went cap in hand to Guide Dogs for the Blind and asked them if they had any puppies that had not made the grade for their training. I knew that the reasons some dogs fail as guide dogs is that they are too inquisitive, too distracted by smells, too lively – and these are the qualities I wanted. I needed dogs who would be assertive enough to demand the attention of their diabetic owners, and who had such a keen sense of smell that they would detect the shifts in blood sugar levels easily and consistently.

The Irish Guide Dogs for the Blind were the first to respond to me. They said if I would give a couple of lectures for them, they would repay me with two dogs. One of those dogs, Lucy, is still with us, working as a cancer-detection dog. To this day, we buy about half of all our puppies that go into training either as assistance dogs or as cancer-detection dogs from Guide Dogs, and we are always grateful to them. In the early days we were even given a puppy by Strathclyde Police, who had a litter from one of their dogs and could spare us one. We are happy to be given suitable dogs, including dogs from rescue centres. It is character and ability that are our two main criteria, and we have become better and better at assessing them. If a dog doesn't make the grade, for whatever reason, we go to great lengths to rehome it with a suitable owner. Our puppies are usually ready to start training, for either bio-detection work or as assistance dogs, from about twelve months old, but naturally some take longer to mature, and may not be ready until sixteen months or so.

A really important development for the future of the charity was when Simone came on board officially.

When she was working at Hearing Dogs she covered a job in the HR department, found she loved the work, and took a college course to qualify in it. She left Hearing Dogs to work in HR for a technology company, leaving when she had her first son, my nephew Jude. She worked part-time until Cameron was born two years later, and that's when she started helping me out, placing the samples for me and recording results. Eventually she was doing so much work for us that her involvement was crucial to the charity and we persuaded her to join the staff.

She came into her own when we started fundraising in earnest. We did our first applications for funding from a desk in her conservatory, writing to a list of about a hundred potential donors, and putting in applications for grants, literally running to the post office to hit deadlines for applications. She wrote thank-you letters, and helped me out when I went to give demonstrations. Her role really grew, and she came on the staff properly when the diabetes-alert work started. Simone is a great people person, and she's the perfect choice to liaise with the clients who need assistance dogs. As her children have grown so have her hours, so that today she is working very nearly full-time as our client support manager.

Although she's not directly involved in training dogs, she and her family live surrounded by them. They now have two dogs: Flint, a fox-red Labrador who is Daisy's nephew, who functions as a quality control dog in the diabetes work, trained to alert to low blood sugars but not destined to be rehomed with a family. He has a vital role in the studies we do to monitor our medical alert work.

She and her family have also adopted a little crossbreed terrier, Luna, whose owners couldn't cope with her – she got her name because the day the owners signed her over was the day of a 'blue moon', which only happens every two or three years.

I've never found it a problem having one of my family working with me. If you ask any of the others who work here, they will tell you I treat Simone the same as any-one else. But we are very in tune with each other, which makes life easier, as I don't have to explain myself to her.

In the early days of the medical assistance work, which took off rapidly, Rob and I both worked train-ing the dogs, with Simone placing them with clients. It was a case of all mixing in together. The one thing that surprised us more than any other (although we should have been expecting it) was just how easy it is to get the dogs to recognise the smell of a diabetes hypo or hyper – that is, when the blood sugar drops too low or rises too high. In those early days we did more training in the clients' homes than we do now: like everything else, we've refined our methods.

Even more surprising, and less predictably so, was the discovery that the dogs' ability to alert increased the longer they were with their client. In all other dog training, when the dog is transferred from the trainer to the client there tends to be a reduction in the dog's performance, probably because the longer the client has the dog, the more relaxed they become in keeping up the training, which needs to be constantly reinforced. It gets diluted, and the performance of the dog drops. For instance, if I trained a gun dog for someone, when I went to check on their partnership a month or so later I invariably found the dog was not working at quite the same high level as it had been for me.

But our Diabetes Alert Dogs get better and better. When one of our training team visits them to see how they are getting on, they find the dog is working at a higher level than when he left us. I've thought about the reason a lot, and have come up with two theories. The first is that because dogs have been genetically selected to live in a pack with us and they have an instinct to protect the pack, at some level they understand that erratic blood sugars are a threat to the wellbeing of the pack.

My second theory is more sinister. Further back in evolution, when they were hunting on plains and selecting other animals as prey, they developed a great ability to know which animal is weaker and easier to capture, even if the animal looked perfectly healthy. The smell of disease may have been a significant pointer in their choice of prey, so they are highly attuned to it.

The answer is probably a combination of the two: an acute ability to smell disease, coupled with a desire to protect the member of their pack who needs it.

Whatever the reason, it was clear that the diabetes assistance training was a success. This not only had the potential to be of enormous benefit to others but also helped our charity to establish itself too. The publicity about Zeta and our first few diabetes dogs was hugely beneficial to our funding and to our profile, and it led to media coverage that really put us on the map.

Lawrence McGinty, the science and medical editor of *ITV News*, came to film at our rickety premises, watching the dogs finding the cancer samples. Now retired, Lawrence is a very well-respected and serious medical journalist, and the fact that he took such an interest in us, despite the persisting scepticism of the medical profession, was a huge vote of confidence for us. He concluded his broadcast by saying that, after fifty days' training, 'I tell you, these dogs really *can* sniff out cancer.'

I said on film: 'If we can work out what the odour of cancer is that the dogs can detect, then potentially in ten to fifteen years' time an electronic nose will be able to do it.'

I have never ruled out the possibility that, ultimately, scientists will devise an electronic system for detecting the odour that is as effective as our dogs are, but as I write this, seven years after Lawrence's broadcast, the dogs are still way ahead of the field. There are electronic noses in existence, but they take far longer and are far less able to detect small amounts of odour. The work, of course, goes on, and I don't dismiss the idea of the electronic nose one day taking over. But I think I was optimistic in my forecast of ten to fifteen years.

Although the charity was becoming more known and established, we were still desperate for funds. People assume that because you have appeared on television, money must be rolling in. It wasn't: Simone, Dad and I spent a lot of time phoning around to various foundations and trusts, virtually begging for help. It was a donation from a local trust fund that enabled us to take on more staff. Pam Jones joined us, manning the office, transporting dogs, looking after our volunteers. We also took on Kimberly Cox, a dog trainer in the local area who Rob knew, and who was ideally suited to work with us because she is, herself, a Type 1 diabetic. Just what we needed! We've used samples of her odour to train our dogs to recognise the distinct smells of hypos and hypers, although the dogs are ultimately trained on the specific smell of their new owners. It means she understands the problems of our diabetic clients, and she's able to put the nervous ones at ease by talking about her own condition. She now heads up the training of our puppies for the medical alert work.

Our medical assistance trainers are a very special band of people. After working long hours training dogs at the charity all day, they set alarm clocks to wake themselves up during the night to give the dogs the opportunity to smell diabetes samples at all hours. Alerting clients at night is an important part of the dogs' work: sometimes a client will recognise their own symptoms during the

day, but not at night (small children usually cannot recognise their symptoms at any time). Waking at night is
no problem for dogs because they have a polyphasic sleep
pattern: they have several sleeps every twenty-four hours,
and waking up in the night means nothing to them.
It's the same response dog owners get when someone
breaks into their house in the middle of the night: the
dog barks and wakes them up. The dog is responding to
the stimulus: in the case of the break-in it's noise, in the
case of a diabetes crisis it's odour. It is such a credit to our
trainers that they are prepared to disturb their own sleep
to help the dogs learn.

From the very beginning of our work in 2008, we
couldn't have survived without the volunteers who
have rallied around us. I made a decision very early
on that none of our dogs would live in kennels. That
was easy when it was a matter of Rob and I training
our own dogs to do cancer-detection work. But with a
much bigger programme of training dogs to go out into
the community to work with people with diabetes (and
later with other life-threatening conditions) we needed
a swelling battalion of volunteers to take the dogs into
their homes, fostering them and helping socialise them.
During the day they come to us for training, but in the
evenings and at weekends, they stay with their foster
carers. As our cancer work has grown we have a lot
more working dogs and dogs in training, and these, too,
live with foster carers.

It is one of my most cherished tenets that dogs flourish better when they are in close contact with human beings who love them. I have seen kennels all over the world, including state-of-the-art ones which have cost millions of pounds. But no matter how well furnished the kennels are, with heated floors and comfy raised beds, dogs prefer to be with people. I don't condemn people who occasionally have to put their dogs into kennels, but I did not want our dogs to be kept there full-time. Other charities do have kennels, and I'm not criticising them, but it's not something I want here. All dogs want is to come out of their cages and sit with a person, and that's a relationship we foster. It especially applies to the type of dogs we train as medical alert dogs: to succeed they have to want to be with their owner, putting their head on the owner's lap, watching them constantly to know when they need help.

From the very beginning, I wanted to make it clear to everyone who came in contact with us that these are loved dogs, that we have a mutual relationship with them, that we are learning from each other and that we treat each other with respect. When I was at university I learned how stroking dogs reduced blood pressure and heart rate in the old and sick, but I also learned that the dogs, too, had better blood pressure and slower heart rates after being petted. It's a two-way relationship.

We support the volunteer carers by paying vets' fees and providing food: from very early on we have been very lucky to have been sponsored by Royal Canin dog food, who generously supply us with all the food we need. Some of our volunteers drop their doggy friends off with us in the morning and pick them up in the afternoon when they have finished their 'work', but others are brought in by members of our staff or other volunteers who do a dog run, in much the same way that parents do a school run. In fact, the hours are very similar: the dogs arrive with us at about 9 am and go home about 3.30 pm. We have four registered volunteer drivers, and their help is vital: we'd lose a precious four hours a day collecting dogs without them.

The dogs are not 'working' all day. Each dog works for three or four twenty-minute sessions. The rest of the time they are out in the field next to our premises being exercised, or loafing around the building. This has got to be one of the few offices where you have to turf a dog off your chair in order to sit down at your computer. If you didn't like dogs, you couldn't work here. On any given day there may be ten dogs in the cancer-detection section, and more in the medical assistance training department.

It has been an organic growth. As our workload has increased, so has the publicity about it, and consequently more volunteers have come forward. But in those early days we needed just a handful of recruits, as well as more to help out in the offices and collect money for us, and we've never been disappointed by their enthusiasm and willingness to do whatever they can to help us.

Richard, my reporter friend, probably came to regret his support of our work – especially after one evening when he and I shared half a bottle of wine, and came up with the hare-brained scheme that we would jump out of a plane to raise funds. Rob and Simone were roped in, and all four of us did a skydive that raised £2,500. It was a beautiful sunny day when we did it, and after initial worries I enjoyed it. I had to ask my GP for a letter allowing me to do it because of my medication, and he said: 'Well, it's not normal for a doctor to approve someone with acute depression jumping out of a plane, but . . .'

We never turned down an invitation to speak and demonstrate with one of our dogs. Rob Harris and I split the requests between us, going to every organisation from Beaver Scout groups to Women's Institutes. We worked weekends and several evenings of the week. We still try to go to any group that wants us, but we have more staff now and there are others, including volunteers who have attended sessions to help them become speakers on our behalf, who share the load. Back then, we saw every invitation as a chance to raise a bit more money, and even after his son Jamie was born in 2011, Rob was willing to turn out. He says, and so do many of the staff here, that this is not just a job, it's a crusade – and one to which we are all passionately committed.

I've always taken on the lion's share of the television, radio, newspaper and magazine publicity work. Every article or film about us generates more support, but also more awareness, which is vital. I've appeared on TV across the world, and although filming always seems to take up a disproportionate amount of time for a few minutes' broadcast, it's worth it if it increases our profile and brings more donors in. Again, I have learned to separate myself from the public appearance: if I am there to talk about the dogs, my passion and enthusiasm takes over, and I don't feel self-conscious or aware that viewers are looking at me. I concentrate on the dogs, and getting my message across.

But while my working life was becoming more and more exciting and satisfying, I was still coping with a legion of problems in my private life, struggling to get the canal cottage into shape to sell it, having run out of money to employ people to help me.

Roger Mugford, who I met when I was at university, came to the first meeting at which we decided to set up the charity and he is now a much-valued advisor and a good friend. When I split with Andy, we had two horses, Harry and Milly. I couldn't live at the cottage and I was away so much, travelling to Korea, so I had to pay livery costs on top of funding the work on the cottage. Roger simply said, 'I'll pick up one of your horses and bring him here. There's a field on the farm he can live in.' It was a very generous offer, and Harry moved there. I managed to find other riders to share the cost of Milly, and after a time Gill Lacey found a home where Harry could go on loan. That's where he was when Andy abruptly demanded a horse back, so that he could sell it. He took Harry, and fortunately the people who were looking after him on loan were willing to buy him.

I still have Milly. She's aged twenty now, and lives in a retirement home: she can't be ridden because of a leg injury, but I try to visit her regularly.

Roger also helped me meet a new friend who was to make a real difference to my social life. He and I travelled to Birmingham for a one-day conference on dog training, stopping on the A1 near Bedford to pick up a young woman, Wendy, who worked for him occasionally, and who was going to the same event. She became a friend, taking me under her wing when she saw that I was still recovering from my deep depression, and that my social life was, at this stage, non-existent. I filled my life with work and my family, but was still very insecure and unhappy. Weekends were hard, when everyone else was busy with their partners and families.

Wendy invited me to a couple of music events: her then husband writes music. One of my great solaces throughout that desperate time was soulful house music, which I have always loved, and I rank music as the third element in my recovery, along with my dogs and my family. My therapist told me to accept invitations, not to become a recluse, and to be open to new experiences. So when my friend invited me to a birthday party in her local village hall, I decided to go, even though it was very tempting to stay home and curl up with Woody. I had no enthusiasm for putting on my makeup and a decent dress, but I forced myself.

The music at the party was great, and I danced all evening, particularly with one guy. He told me he was single and he chatted me up in breaks from dancing.

'I'm not looking for a boyfriend,' I said, sincerely. I really did not want to plunge into another relationship.

'Would you like me to show you Bedford?'

'No. No . . .' I said, suppressing a smile at this unusual chat-up line.

'What's your favourite place in Britain?'

'Dorset,' I replied, without thinking.

'Right, how about we go down to Dorset for a weekend?'

'No, I'm not in the right place to go anywhere with anyone . . .'

At the end of the party a group of us were going back to my friend's cottage for coffee. I'd been invited to stay the night, and my dancing companion came too. As we were walking along the corridor to leave the hall, he said: 'I really would like to take you out.'

As soon as he said it a loud voice from behind us said: 'I don't think your wife would like that.'

My dance partner responded: 'F*** off, mate,' to the man who had made the remark.

'Are you married?' I asked.

'I was . . .'

Then the same voice interrupted. 'No, you *are* married. You've got five children.'

My dance partner turned, looking as though he would punch the man behind, who calmly put his hand on his friend's shoulder and said: 'I'll get my car and give you a lift.'

I'm a bit of a petrol head, and I looked in admiration at this man's shiny Audi TT, which was race modified. He dropped his mate home, presumably to his wife and five children, and then joined us at my friend's cottage for coffee. I learned that he wrote music with my friend's husband. We talked for quite a time, mostly about sat-navs. Eventually he told me he is a carpenter, and that his name is Rob.

I met him two or three more times, at music events and at my friend's cottage. We chatted a lot, but it was very gentle, and there was no pressure from him. I was trying to do what the Korean teller had told me: go with the flow of the water, don't fight against it. Eventually I was invited by Wendy to a New Year's Eve party, and she said: 'Rob will be there.'

'Is that the carpenter?'

'Yes, he's really keen on you. We've known him for years and we've never seen him keen on anyone before. He's a good guy. He asked if you will be coming.'

'There will never be anything between us,' I said. 'I'm not in the right place.'

During the evening she made sure I was alone with Rob, and at one point he said, 'Can I ask you something? Why have you got a big wall around you?'

I told him I had been badly hurt.

'Well, hiding behind a wall isn't going to make it better.'

'I'm trying, but it's very hard. The hurt was very deep.'

We talked and I found that he had been really badly wounded by a difficult childhood. He also made me a great offer: 'If you make me dinner, I'll have a look at your house and we can start getting it back to how it should be.'

I didn't commit. But as a group of us walked back after midnight he said again: 'Can I come and help you?'

As he said it, I looked up. It was a crisp night with a large moon, and I saw a white feather, bright in the moonlight, spiralling down from a great height. It was eerie: where could it come from at that time of night? I watched it until it landed at my feet. Wendy picked it up and handed it to me: 'Claire, that's for you.'

In that moment I made a decision: it was a new year, the Korean teller had told me not to fight the current, my therapist told me to be open to new experiences, and on a very practical level I needed all the help I could get.

'Yes, you can help me,' I said.

After that, Rob came every weekend and worked very hard, turning the cottage from a gutted shell into a lovely home that eventually I could sell. Andy was sending me solicitor's letters accusing me of obstructing the sale, but I ignored them because he had taken no interest and had no idea what a bad state it had been in. Rob and I worked side by side with him doing all the structural work, installing a kitchen, and me wielding a paintbrush.

We didn't embark on a relationship straightaway. Whenever he asked me out, I rejected him. It wasn't because I didn't like him, but it took me a long time to feel safe enough to commit. It was only later, with hindsight, that I remembered the teller's prediction that I would meet a man who was younger than me, not what I was looking for, and that I would reject him several times.

Although Rob's background and his work is very different from mine, he has been a steady and reliable influence on me since he first came into my life. And I was about to need his calm support, and that of my amazing family, more than ever.

CHAPTER NINE

Daisy Saves my Life

'Come on, Daisy, out you get.'

For the first time ever, Daisy was reluctant to leap out of the boot of my car for a run with the other dogs, Tangle and Woody, and another little dog I was looking after that day. When I opened the boot, Tangle took a flying leap out and was already snuffling around in the vegetation, with the little dog following him. Woody, who needed to be lifted down, gave his usual excited whimper and waited for me to put him on the ground, immediately scuttling off on his wonky legs in pursuit of the others. But Daisy stood in the boot, nudging my chest with her nose and staring up into my face intently with her big, brown eyes, forcing me to pay attention to her.

'Stop it, Daise,' I said. 'C'mon, don't you want a run?'

The dogs had been cooped up for a while because I'd been to a meeting in Reading. Afterwards, I knew they would be keen to get out into the fresh air and have some exercise, so I stopped at an area of fields and woods to let them run. But Daisy was refusing to leave the boot, and was still pushing her nose into my chest. It was very odd: she was normally as keen and energetic as the others. I gave a quick tug on her collar, and after a backward glance at me she finally jumped down and set off after the other two.

Daisy has always been one of my very special dogs. There is a deep understanding between us, and it is this bond that I believe saved my life.

That evening I noticed that my chest was sore. I thought she had bruised it with her persistent nudging. But when I rubbed it I detected a small lump in one of my breasts. I wasn't too worried: it was very tiny, and I had read that most breast lumps are benign. But my sister, Louise, a doctor, insisted that I see my GP.

'I can't – I've got too much work on, and I'm due to go away.'

'Claire, make the appointment *now*.'

My GP reassured me that the lump was probably nothing to worry about, but said I had to go to a specialist breast cancer clinic for a proper diagnosis. I repeated what I said to Louise: 'I'm too busy – can I go in two or three weeks?'

'No, you should never be too busy for your health.'

So off I went a couple of days later and had a biopsy and a mammogram. When I went back for the results the specialist said: 'The good news is that your biopsy results are clear, the lump is a benign cyst. But there is something showing up on your mammogram, much deeper than this lump. We want to do a core biopsy.'

He explained I would have to go to another hospital for this procedure. When I went for the appointment the nurse told me how long it would take, but it actually took a lot longer, and I had to have extra injections of local anaesthetic. She apologised for it taking so long, saying that the consultant was clearly being very thorough.

I had to return a few days later for the result, and this time Mum and Dad, who had been with me to all my appointments, weren't able to come. I said I would drive myself, but they were worried about me being on my own. Although, at this stage, I thought I was coping OK with all the tests, a strange thing happened: I started falling asleep during the day. I've never been able to sleep easily, and have always struggled on planes and even in my own bed to get off to sleep. But now I even missed a station when I was on a train because I nodded off.

This increased Mum and Dad's anxiety, so they were relieved when I told them that Rob had a day off work and would drive me. He had only been my boyfriend for a couple of months, although he had been a really good friend for over six months. To my surprise, when we got to the hospital he volunteered to come into the appointment with me, which I appreciated.

When the consultant came into the room he was accompanied by a nurse. I feared the worst: I'd heard somewhere that doctors like to have a nurse sitting with you when they break the news that you have cancer. Whether it's true or not as a general rule, it was for me.

'We have found it early, and we'll operate within a few days,' the doctor said. He explained that I had a breast cancer tumour that was very deep, and then listed in fairly rapid succession what would happen next. He said he hoped I would only need a lumpectomy, an operation to remove the lump and some tissue around it; sentinel lymph nodes would be removed to test whether the cancer had spread; with luck I would not need chemotherapy but would definitely need to have radiotherapy, which would last a few weeks. He said the operation would take place in a few days' time.

As he listed each thing, I heard a sharp intake of breath from Rob, and when I looked at him he had gone very white – so much so that the cancer nurse asked him if he was all right. He was more shocked and upset than I was.

Because I was so low, still in the throes of depression, I don't think I reacted in the way most people do when they are given a cancer diagnosis. I assumed it was probably a death sentence because I knew nothing about the treatment and the prognosis, and the word 'cancer' seemed to spell doom. But I was strangely calm. I felt I had lost my husband, and I was desperately trying to plough on through a rotten life, and if this was going to be the end, maybe that was the best thing that could happen. I was struggling to keep my head above water with all the problems I had, and now I didn't want to struggle any more.

Several years earlier, when I was happy with Andy, I remember thinking that the one thing I really did not want to have was breast cancer, because I had all the familiar fears about it disfiguring my body, and being a threat to my identity as a woman. But now, I felt I didn't care. In the days before the operation, I thought: 'I've lost my soul mate, so it doesn't matter what I look like. And if I'm going to pop my clogs, it will be the answer to everything.'

I even pathetically hoped at first that when Andy heard of my illness he would come rushing back to me, but I was soon disillusioned about that: I never heard anything personal from him, he showed no concern for me despite all the years we had been together.

I couldn't work out how I could fit in the treatment, while I was still trying to get the house ready to sell, and while my savings from the Samsung work were dwindling so fast that I would not have any money to live on very soon if I didn't work. There was a deep feeling of despair. I felt I was going to go into bankruptcy, the house would be left to decay. My God, I can't do all this ...

Life was much more daunting to me than death, at that time.

Of course, my brain was not computing how much help I would have from everyone who rallied around me. Mum and Dad completely supported me. Rob, who must have wondered what he'd got himself into, remained steadfast and carried on working on the house, as well as driving me all over the place. And when I curled up with Woody snuggled against me, I realised I could not possibly leave him. Who else would understand his funny little ways? Who else would know when he needed to be picked up, wanted to be put down? Who else would respond to his strange little scream for help?

Because I was in this weird frame of mind, I didn't worry as much about the operation as I probably would have done normally. My fear of needles and the whole hospital process was overpowered by my depression, and I felt resigned rather than fearful.

Thankfully, the operation was a success, and I was told afterwards that my cancer was so deep that by the time I had been able to feel it, it would almost certainly have been too late.

'If you hadn't come in for a check-up . . .'

As the consultant said the words, I remembered Daisy nudging me, I could see the pleading look in her eyes, and I knew that, without her, I was unlikely to have ever noticed the small benign lump that led to the much deeper cancer being caught. She had saved my life. I had joined the large pool of dog owners who had been alerted to serious conditions by their pets. And it's not only dogs that do it: there are stories of cats and other animals. John Church, who collects all this anecdotal evidence, even knows of a parrot who alerted his owner that there was something wrong.

The sentinel lymph nodes that were removed from under my arm were clear, which meant the cancer had not spread, and I did not need chemotherapy, which is like winning the breast-cancer lottery. I had a numb arm for some years afterwards, caused by the removal of the nodes, which affected me riding a horse and even walking a dog on a lead, but that is a small price to pay.

I decided against having reconstruction surgery. At the time, my self-esteem was so low it didn't seem important. Rob told me immediately that it made no difference to him, which boosted my confidence, because it is a disfiguring operation. I'm sure many men, if they'd only been going out with someone for a couple of months, would have run for the hills with everything I loaded on to him, but he was very straightforward and has never seen it as an issue. I call myself 'one and a half boobs', and the only time I've been self-conscious about it, and regretted not having the reconstruction, was when I was at a pool party surrounded by women who had clearly had breast enlargements.

After the operation I was referred to Alan Makepeace, an oncologist at Mount Vernon Hospital in Hertfordshire, who organised my radiotherapy. He admits he was sceptical about my story of Daisy finding my cancer, although he had heard other stories about the ability of animals to pick up on disease. But I talked with such conviction about my work that he agreed to come and see the dogs, and now both he and my surgeon are great supporters of MDD.

Like everyone who sees the dogs working, Alan was moved as he watched them unerringly identifying the samples from patients with cancer. But he stresses that it is the solid scientific basis of our work that completely convinced him, the fact that everything is tested robustly. He says that he is immensely impressed by my dedication to scientific methods, and the fact that I am not simply an enthusiast with a collection of anecdotal evidence.

'When I first saw the dogs working I was won over, as most people are.'

So having cancer brought me two more supporters, and from the medical profession, too. But it was a high price to pay. I found the radiotherapy gruelling. The routine of going to Mount Vernon five times a week for four weeks really took it out of me, and I found the drug I was supposed to take for five years caused so many side effects that after two years I stopped taking it.

My divorce from Andy came through just as my radiotherapy treatment was finally over, although it did not bring the closure everyone predicted, and I was still very raw and emotionally battered by it all.

I believe the theory that stress can cause or exacerbate cancer. In 2012, research scientists at UCLA published a study that showed toxic relationships can lead to illnesses ranging from high blood pressure to heart disease and cancer. My body was reacting to my deep depression, and the hassle I was having with the house renovations. It was all too much, and cancer was the outcome. The Koreans have long accepted that trauma causes physical ill health, and it is now being accepted much more in the Western world. There are many stories of people – and dogs – dying from a broken heart, and I accept these are true, too, and that there will one day be a scientific explanation of how unhappiness and trauma can lead to physical illness and death.

Thankfully, when the radiotherapy treatment was over, I recovered pretty well, apart from the side effects of the drug regime. There was a residual tiredness, but before too long I was back to working long hours, especially as we were now getting into high gear with our diabetes-alert dogs. I had very little social life, filling my diary with speaking engagements and demonstrations, mainly to bring in more funding, but also to stop me thinking about my failed marriage.

CHAPTER TEN

Sleep at Night

I have never doubted that we were right to expand from cancer detection into providing alert dogs, and every time I look around the office, I'm reinforced in that decision. There are always puppies and young dogs around, being trained to recognise the smells of disease, and waiting, though they don't know it, to be partnered with someone whose life they will change, even save.

Placing dogs with families with children is one of the most moving parts of alert work. We see families where the parents are on their knees with tiredness, working together in shifts to get up through the night to test their child's blood, then having to look after other children, go to work and get through a normal day. They spend hours sitting by hospital beds when their child collapses, and the strain and worry is etched on their faces when they come to us.

The joy that a dog can bring to families near break-ing point is worth all the work and struggle to raise funds that we face. I had no idea what it was like living with a small child who was so dangerously ill before I met some of our clients. I remember clearly talking to Debbie Davies, who had to give up her job as a teacher to become a full-time carer for her two-year-old daughter Cerys, when Cerys was diagnosed with Type 1 diabetes. Her husband, Hywel, also took three months off work: waking up every two hours during the night, every night, to test Cerys's blood sugar levels took a huge toll on both her parents, with a knock-on effect on their two older children, Erin and Rhys. It was a very rocky time for the whole family.

'We didn't sleep, it was hellish,' Debbie told me. 'We were surviving, not living, and all we were doing was keeping Cerys alive. We were lurching from crisis to crisis every day. We were ragged from lack of sleep and our whole family was suffering.'

Cerys was so sensitive to insulin that life revolved around checking her levels, with her sleeping in her parents' bed so that they could test her every hour or two hours through the night, their lives dominated by the tyranny of the alarm clock. When Debbie first contacted us, she was disappointed to be told that Cerys was too young for a dog, but nevertheless she was inspired by our work and hopeful that one day this would be the answer for Cerys. Debbie's sister and brother-in-law launched an ambitious programme of fundraising events for us and through them Debbie was invited to one of our open days.

In Debbie's words: 'I cried when I heard Claire talking at the open day about what the dogs can do. I immediately knew she got it: she understands it, she knows what it was like to live like us.'

Although Cerys was not quite five at this stage, after talking to Debbie that day I promised to have a look at her application, because I could see what a struggle they were having. I talked to Simone and Kimberly, and we decided to put Cerys forward for a dog.

Simone made the phone call to Debbie to tell her the news. As Debbie describes it: 'We were on holiday in Abersoch in Wales; it was pouring with rain and I was shopping in Asda. I dropped my bags – everything went everywhere. I was so thrilled by the news, I couldn't speak.'

It was a big decision for the family: Debbie was frightened of dogs after a childhood incident, and Hywel grew up on a farm with working dogs who were never allowed in the house.

But when a black Labrador called Wendy bounded into their lives, tail wagging and nose sniffing the air, ever alert for changes in Cerys's sugar levels, she gave them back their lives. As Debbie says: 'It was like a miracle had come into the house, a snuffly wet-nosed miracle.'

Wendy is Cerys's personal medical attendant, sleeping next to her bed, and getting up through the night to wake Debbie or Hywel if Cerys's levels are moving away from the norm. She alerts them two or three times a week – a huge, life-changing difference for them, and one that has brought family life back to a happy normality.

Wendy's skills are extraordinary. Cerys goes to football training with her older sister Erin, and Hywel coaches the team. From the touchline, Wendy has alerted him to Cerys's blood sugar levels moving out of safe levels. At home she has alerted from downstairs when Cerys was playing upstairs. Again, I'll leave it to Debbie to explain the impact it has had on their lives:

The whole team at Medical Detection Dogs worked with me to give me confidence. They had to find a dog that was good with little children, very gentle, but also confident enough and forceful enough to wake us up if Cerys needs us. We are different people now that we can sleep again, and Cerys is delighted with her companion.

Wendy is Cerys's guardian angel, she sees her role as looking after Cerys. She came to get me one night when Cerys was having a nosebleed, nothing to do with her diabetes. And another time she fetched me because Cerys was crying after an argument with her brother . . .

When Cerys was very poorly and had to stay in hospital, Wendy slept by her bed there, and alerted. She goes to the diabetes clinic with us, where everyone loves her. Cerys's HbA1c [glycated haemoglobin] levels have improved so much since we've had Wendy, and we know this will make a huge impact on her future life. We could not get those levels without a dog, because Wendy alerts so early, as the blood sugars are just starting to change.

The savings to the NHS are incalculable, both now and in the future for Cerys. We are both so grateful and in awe of what Claire has done: she had a vision and she has pushed it through, despite all the obstacles and scepticism. She and her whole team are miracle workers.

MDD go to amazing lengths to make sure everything is working well. Kimberly even came to our house to teach Wendy not to chase our cats!

There are so many amazing stories: a teenager who has been able to go to her first sleepover, and to the cinema without her parents (the dog sleeps through the films!); another who has been able to leave home to go to college, which she never thought would be possible; a dog who splits his time alerting for a father and his young son, who both have diabetes.

When I talk to our grateful clients, I am constantly moved to tears, and very proud of the work we do.

When we started training diabetes-alert dogs, we followed the model that I had established with Zeta and Cherry, moving into the clients' homes to train the dogs. But we soon realised that the demand was huge, and to even begin to fulfil it we had to find a way to do it more efficiently. We puzzled over it, and then hit on the idea of getting the diabetic clients to breathe on to swabs when their blood sugar levels were out of kilter, then to freeze the swabs and send them to us. In those early days, Simone and I chopped up cotton sheets to make the swabs, carefully handling them with surgical gloves on, and providing pots for them to be stored in.

It was remarkably successful. We found that we could train the dogs with the samples, so that by the time the clients came to spend a week with us at the centre, the dogs were already familiar with their odours, and knew them as if they had seen a photograph. Our system now is that we choose our clients on the basis of their need: those with the greatest need may wait a shorter time for a dog than others. We have a waiting list of up to three years for dogs. By the end of 2015, we had seventy dogs working in the community, five in training and more than forty at the puppy-walking stage. We are trying to increase the numbers, so that we will be able to offer dogs to thirty-four clients a year, but of course everything depends on funding. It costs approximately £12,000 to train an alert dog, and when you look at the amount that saves the NHS in the ten years or so that each dog looks after their owner, it's very cheap at the price. Each time a dog prevents an ambulance call-out, it saves £250, and each time it prevents an overnight stay in hospital, it save £1,700. If a dog alerts three or four times a day, as is often the case for our clients with diabetes over a working life of up to ten years – well, the potential sum saved runs into millions, and is multiplied by the number of clients we have.

We know that it saves hospital admissions, when the patient has a diabetic crisis; we know the dogs keep people in work and independent; we know there are tremendous psychological rewards. What we don't know yet, but will learn over the next few years, is to what extent the dogs help our clients avoid some of the worst, long-term side effects of diabetes, including blindness, cardiovascular disease, kidney failure and loss of sensation in feet, which can, in extreme cases, lead to amputation. Our clients report that their HbA1c levels are generally very much improved by having a dog that alerts early to blood sugar changes. HbA1c is measured every few months and gives doctors a picture of average blood sugar levels over that period. Good control lowers the risks of complications, and the fact that our dogs alert so early means that our clients report back that their HbA1c levels are better and steadier than they have ever been.

A study of seventeen of our clients done by Dr Nicola Rooney from Bristol University confirmed what we knew: they all reported a decrease in the number of times paramedics were called to them, fewer unconscious episodes and improved independence.

Of course, many people with diabetes have a keen awareness of when their blood sugar levels are out of kilter. But the longer – and better – they monitor their own condition, the more likely it is that one day some of them will lose the ability to recognise the feelings that come before the levels slip into the danger zone, which is what happened with Cherry. He had very poor hypogly-caemic awareness and could not recognise the blood sugar changes in his body. It's a condition that affects 10 per cent of all diabetics.

The other group of people with diabetes who are also unable to recognise the signs that things are sliding out of control are young children, like Cerys.

Rebecca Farrar, aged six at the time, was one of our very first child clients, and we teamed her with a yellow Labrador called Shirley back in 2009. It was so early in our history that we didn't even have our distinctive red coats available at that time. Rebecca had been taken into hos-pital eight times in a critical condition after collapsing, before Shirley came into her life. Again, her mum had needed to give up her job to be on hand at all times, and was catnapping through the night with an alarm clock to wake her to monitor Rebecca's levels regularly. Once Shirley arrived, her mum could sleep, safe in the knowl-edge that Shirley was on duty.

Shirley had been given to us by Guide Dogs because she did not like wearing the necessary harness. But her puppy walker herself had diabetes and she noticed that Shirley licked her hand whenever her blood sugars were out of kilter, so we found it easy to retrain her. Rebecca's school were so impressed by the calm way that Shirley stayed by Rebecca, and alerted by picking up her blood-testing kit, that they asked us if it would be all right for Shirley to go into school every day. We familiarised Shirley with the school environment, and after a bit of fussing and petting from the other children, she now settles down every day by Rebecca's side in class.

Lawrence McGinty from ITV again championed our cause by filming a piece about Rebecca and Shirley in February 2011. It went out on the early evening news bulletin, but by ten o'clock, the main bulletin, we lost our slot because of the heartwarming story of an elderly lady who attacked some young men who were robbing a jeweller's shop, hitting them with her handbag. We were sad to have been dropped, but that's the nature of news – and, even without the later broadcast, Lawrence's report led to me being asked to appear on the *Daybreak* ITV programme, hosted by Adrian Chiles and Christine Bleakley, with Rebecca and Shirley in the studio too. Another great publicity coup which, as well as helping with fundraising, brought in a slew of new applicants to have dogs, in particular from families struggling to look after young children.

One such child was Gemma Faulkner. She was seven when her mum Clare got in touch with us, after reading one of the newspaper articles that arose from the TV coverage. It was another two years before we were able to provide Gemma with a companion, but from that day, Polo, a black Labrador, has completely changed the Faulkners' lives, just as Wendy has for the Davies family. Gemma was also very young when she was diagnosed with Type 1 diabetes, two weeks before her third birthday. It was a very scary time, and the family's whole life was scheduled around trying to keep her well. When she was old enough to go to school, Clare had to go in at lunchtime to give her an injection, which meant she had to give up her job.

Clare admits she wasn't convinced when she read about Rebecca and Shirley. She thought it couldn't possibly be as good as the journalist made out, and she didn't want to raise Gemma's expectations. But she and her husband Julian were exhausted by the relentless schedule of two-hour testing through the night, and they were willing to try anything. During the day, monitoring her condition was not too difficult, but at night Gemma had no awareness of when her blood sugars were dropping or rising.

When Clare contacted us, the family went through our standard application procedure, providing us with supporting evidence from Gemma's specialist paediatric consultant and her diabetes nurse. They also had to record three months of her blood sugar levels. After eighteen months on the waiting list, the Faulkners were interviewed, and then got a date to come to our headquarters to meet up with the team.

Our normal procedure means we introduced Gemma to a couple of dogs who were around that day – one was my dog Daisy. We wanted to see how she got on with them, as the Faulkners didn't have a pet dog, and we needed to feel they were all comfortable around dogs, especially Gemma. In February 2012, they again travelled from their home near Chichester to Buckinghamshire to meet Polo.

There's a very important dynamic between a client and a dog. Simone, who works on this side of the charity and is very involved in matching partnerships, describes it as a spiritual moment when she sees a dog and a potential owner really hit it off. Polo had previously been teamed with two possible clients before he met Gemma, but it had not worked out. Yet the minute he met Gemma it was clear to everyone that the bond was there. Gemma loved him as soon as she saw him.

Many dogs alert parents of children with diabetes by taking the blood-testing kit to them, but Polo was never happy handling the kit, so he has a toy bone that he thrusts into Gemma's mother Clare's face when he needs her to wake up. If she doesn't rouse, he jumps on the bed until either she or Julian go to Gemma. Gemma's parents still have to get up in the night: children's levels can be particularly erratic, especially during growth spurts. But they can relax before and after Polo has woken them, knowing that he is on duty, and instead of getting up four or five times a night to check Gemma's blood sugar levels, it's now only a couple of times a week.

In Clare's words: 'I can honestly say that Polo transformed our lives. We were sleep-deprived, which leads to anxieties, arguments, stress – we were pretty highly strung before Polo came into our family. Gemma's blood levels were a constant preoccupation. We've got our normal lives back, and it's all thanks to a dog.'

Polo goes everywhere with Gemma, and has even taken to kayaking – although he's liable to jump into the water to swim after ducks …

Our clients, the people who have dogs placed with them, are very enthusiastic supporters of our charity, and it's wonderful to see them when they bring their dogs along to support our open days and other events. I never tire of hearing their stories of how having a dog has changed their lives.

Importantly, we don't only train dogs to recognise diabetes. It was soon after the surge of publicity about our first diabetes dogs that I was contacted by Karen Ruddlesden, who has Addison's disease, and asked if I could train a dog for her. We were still in the early days of refining our diabetes training, and when I looked into it I discovered that no dog had ever been trained to detect Addison's.

The first thing I had to do was find out about the disease, and assess whether I thought it would have a smell that a dog could pick up on. Addison's disease occurs when the adrenal glands are not functioning properly: in Karen's case, tumours on her adrenal glands led to them being removed completely in order to save her life. Without them, though, her body is dangerously low in cortisol and aldosterone, and in order to compensate Karen was on a high dose of steroids all the time.

People with Addison's disease can suffer sudden drops in cortisol levels, which cause dizziness, fainting, vomiting and cramps, and Karen had been rushed to hospital many times after collapsing.

I knew that anecdotally dogs can smell fear, which causes raised levels of cortisol, and cortisol can also be measured in saliva. So it seemed to make sense that the smell of cortisol, and the changing levels of it, would be there on the breath of the Addison's patient. We set about looking for a dog to train, knowing that it would have be a special, extra-confident dog to rouse Karen when she was slipping into a coma.

Kimberly had only recently started working with us, and she said: 'I think I've got a dog we can train for Addison's. He's a chocolate Lab, very full of himself, a bit out of control, and his owners don't think they can keep him because he's wrecking their house . . .'

My mind went straight back to Ruffles, who had come to me in very similar circumstances.

It may not sound sensible that a dog who is out of control will make a good alert dog, but, as with Ruffles, he was clearly a very intelligent dog who simply wasn't getting enough stimulation. We knew that we needed a very confident dog, a dog that could problem-solve in stressful situations, a dog that would not be distressed if he found himself surrounded by paramedics after his owner had gone into a crisis.

Kimberly and I went to see Coco, and were back at the headquarters discussing whether he was right for the Addison's training when the owners rang up and said we either took him straightaway or he went to a rescue centre, as he was chewing everything, running away, and they couldn't cope. Kimberly brought him in.

'I think he's all right. He's bomb proof – nothing bothers him.'

As she said this, she was towed into my office by him as if she were on skis, and he promptly knocked about four things over. He was a hooligan, but I'd much rather start work with a hooligan than with a dog who is too timid, and with Karen's acute condition it was very important that he wasn't fazed by anything. He was clearly very confident, and all his naughty behaviours were because he was bored and trying to entertain himself.

We put him with one of our experienced puppy walkers, who struggled a bit with his wayward behaviour, but who gave him lots of basic training, and slowly a super, confident, bright dog began to emerge. When I was sure he was the right dog, Karen came in to meet him. They immediately fell in love, and she's a strong enough personality to cope with him.

We asked her to take samples of her breath and sweat whenever she was going into an Addisonian crisis, and when the little pots started to arrive from her I trained

Coco to pick up the odour, and then lick her hand and nudge her when he smelled it.

Like so many other clients, Karen's life has been transformed. She takes oral medication when he alerts her, and if that isn't enough, she injects herself. Sometimes she still ends up in hospital.

'But each time I am treated in resus in A&E they tell me that I would not have survived if I hadn't had the early alert,' she told me.

Because of Coco, Karen's preventative levels of steroids have been cut, which makes her feel fitter and more active. She has been able to have holidays, she can go out on her own, she is happier and more confident. She has other health problems, like infections, and Coco visits her in hospital – and immediately checks her breath.

We had a boost when Karen's story was highlighted on the BBC's *Inside Out* programme. The programme started with a dramatic question: if someone saved your life on a daily basis, how would you thank them? After an explanation of Addison's disease, there was a film about Karen and Coco, and Karen explained how Coco paws at her, jumps on the bed, paws her face until she comes round. 'He's my friend, my safeguard, I trust him and he trusts me. He has my life in his paws,' she said.

Gratifyingly, in the face of the scepticism we still faced from many medics, Karen's doctor spoke publicly on television about the amazing benefits that Coco brings, explaining that the dog can detect changes in her cortisol levels far more quickly and efficiently than any medical test, and because Karen's condition changes so quickly, her life would be in constant danger without Coco.

A great highlight for Karen and Coco came when they were nominated to carry the Olympic torch before the London 2012 Olympics. As usual, Coco was delighted with all the attention, and behaved perfectly. Our unruly, out-of-control hooligan was a star.

Since our success with the world's first Addison's dog, we have trained dogs for other specific conditions. We have a dog working in partnership with a client with narcolepsy, and we have a dog working with a client, Sam Sutcliffe, who has POTS (postural orthostatic tachycardia syndrome). This is a condition which causes sudden surges in heartbeat and a drop in blood pressure, which can lead to dizziness and fainting. Sam was frequently collapsing, as often as three times a day, and could be unconscious for anything from a minute to an hour. She ran the risk of damaging herself every time she fell, and her life was one of constant fear. But with a dog alerting her, she has time to make sure she is sitting or lying in a secure place. There is no cure for POTS, but her medical alert dog has made her feel much safer, and she is able to go out more. We are not sure how the dog detects it, although I believe it is an odour change because we trained the dog with breath and sweat samples obtained for us by someone else when she was collapsed.

New knowledge is being amassed all the time, and we are constantly learning more about what dogs are capable of. Tony Robinson's Jack Russell cross terrier, Ssafa, named after the military charity, was already alerting Tony when he got in contact with us. Tony, who served for many years in the armed forces, has a debilitating condition, acute spondylitis and arthritis, which means he is in a wheelchair. He suffers from sudden, sharp attacks of debilitating pain, for which he needs to take morphine. Tony and his family noticed that Ssafa started behaving oddly about an hour before the pain attacks. They carefully logged the times and dates. By chance, Tony met one of our trainers at a show where we had a stand, and talked about what was going on.

I was intrigued: here we had a little dog who was doing instinctively what we were training dogs to do. I went to see Tony at home, and then he started a training programme under Rob Harris to refine Ssafa's alert behaviour, and to allow her to wear one of our distinctive red coats, enabling Tony to take her with him to places where dogs are not normally allowed. When Ssafa alerts, Tony takes extra medication, which means he does not have to be rushed to A&E in a crisis.

Another challenge we faced was helping a woman who is severely allergic to nuts. We had worked with nut allergies before, and had trained dogs to sniff out nuts in food, and to alert if there was the smell of nuts on a chair or other surface. Someone who has handled nuts can leave a trace on a chair that, if touched by the person with the nut allergy, can be transferred to them and ingested through their eyes if they touch their face. Training a dog for this work was an extension of what we were already doing. But when this client, Tara, got in touch, she explained that her condition is much more severe: she reacts to airborne allergens, and is at risk of going into anaphylactic shock if there is a trace of nuts in the air in a room where they have been eaten the day before, or if they are on the breath of someone who had a peanut-butter sandwich the previous day, even if they have cleaned their teeth in between. Her level of sensitivity is something I had never encountered before.

Again, we had to train the dog counter-intuitively. A normal nut-allergy dog will save its owner from touching or eating a sandwich containing nuts by scratching and showing them the offending item. With Tara and her dog Willow, we needed a dog to do the opposite from showing, to take her away from any slight trace of nuts in the air. The challenge was to get a dog to recognise such slight odours, and to then remove her from danger. We managed it, and Tara is now much happier about going out on her own.

I am always happy to take on a new challenge, and whenever we get asked to look at helping someone with a condition we have never encountered, we are finding that we can almost always help. As I am constantly saying, I don't think we have started to tap into the huge resource that is a dog's nose . . .

CHAPTER ELEVEN

By Royal Appointment

'Good God, quick, get over here and check this out! It's amazing . . .' Actress Lesley Nicol, famous for her role as Mrs Patmore the cook in the hugely successful TV series *Downton Abbey*, was at a dog show near where she was living in West London, when she heard someone shout across to their friends. Lesley, who was strolling around with her two dogs, Bertie and Freddie, decided she had to see what the fuss was about.

She walked across to our stand, where one of our medical assistance dogs, in its bright red coat, was standing with its owner. A volunteer explained all about our work, both in cancer detection and diabetes alerts, and Lesley was immediately struck by it.

'When I heard what MDD was doing a lightbulb went off in my head,' says Lesley, who was appearing in the first series of *Downton* at the time. 'It made sense: everything fell into place. Of course dogs can do these amazing things. The biggest surprise is that it has taken so long for someone to come along and show us all.'

Lesley made contact with us and offered her services to help in any way she could. She came to see a demonstration at an open day, and she not only saw the cancer-detection dogs working, but while she was there she witnessed a dog alerting a client with diabetes to a sugar imbalance.

In her words: 'I learned that the people working at MDD are extraordinary, and the stories of the people they are helping are extraordinary. I couldn't walk away: I wanted to help, whatever I could do.'

We were thrilled to make Lesley an ambassador, and she has been a tremendous boon to us, always promoting us whenever she can, attending Crufts to help man our stand, and being on hand for all the big events we have hosted. She is now living in Hollywood, but still does everything she can to keep our name in the public eye.

We have even named one of our alert dogs Patmore, in honour of Lesley's character. She is a pretty apricot-blonde poodle; Lesley jokes that we have brilliantly matched their hair colour.

Just before Lesley came on board, we moved out of the premises at Westcott into a much more suitable building at Great Horwood, in Buckinghamshire, where we are still based today. We knew we had to move: the Westcott buildings would never have passed the standards laid down by Assistance Dogs International, and if we wanted to be accredited for our work placing dogs with clients with diabetes and other diseases, we had to have better facilities. Besides, it was December 2010 and winter again, and we really did not relish going through another freezing few months.

Once again, we drove around looking at various possible places. Great Horwood is a pretty village north of Milton Keynes, and our headquarters are about a mile outside the village, on a business park (although our building is not part of the business park). Again, one of the main attractions was that there was green space around, where we could exercise the dogs. We were later able to buy a paddock adjoining the site, and enclose it for the dogs.

The building was divided into three units, and we could only afford to rent one. Two of them were empty, and I was tempted to choose the end one, because it had a good entrance for clients. But the middle unit was slightly larger and Dad, sensible as always, pointed out to me that if we were in the middle we would keep our options open for further expansion – good advice, as we now occupy all three units. The building was a shell when we moved in, but we quickly had internal walls installed, giving us a large room to use for the cancer and bio-detection. Instead of a viewing gallery, we had windows in the wall that adjoins the corridor, so that visitors could watch the work.

Life was beginning to get slightly easier, financially, as the charity became more established. Rob, Simone and I were now able to take salaries, and Rob was working full-time. Having finally sold the home I shared with Andy some months earlier, I bought my own house shortly before we moved out of Westcott, so it was a time of upheaval all round. (More recently, in 2015, I have moved again, into a lovely house that I can see myself staying in forever.)

Some of our puppy walkers and volunteers stuck with us through the move: the new headquarters is about twenty-five minutes' drive away from the old building. But we always need more volunteers, and local publicity brings us recruits. Thankfully, we have never been held back in our work by lack of foster homes for our dogs, but we always need more. I am in awe of our puppy trainers and socialisers, because I think it must be so hard to work with a puppy, to train him to the point where he is good to live with, and then hand him over and start again with another one.

It's not just a matter of socialising the puppies in a normal way: our assistance dogs have to be familiar with the insides of shops, schools, cafés, churches, anywhere that their new owners may need to go. The puppies are not allowed to wear our special coats until they are fully trained, but when they start going out and about we give them a lead slip that shows they are in training.

Among all the many people I owe thanks to are the local supermarkets, shops, the bowling alley and restaurants in and around Milton Keynes who allow our puppies in. They are not legally obliged to do so until the dogs are with the clients they care for, but it's a chicken-and-egg situation: it's vital we take the dogs into places the clients need to go, otherwise they will never learn and won't be sufficiently trained for us to hand them over. We are all grateful that we have a good support network of local businesses who are happy to help. I also really appreciate the supporters who don't live near enough to help out with fostering, but give us financial support, paying to keep one of our puppies in training.

As well as our wonderful puppy walkers, we have permanent foster carers for the bio-detection dogs who work on cancer detection: at least they have the dog forever, and he lives with them for the rest of his life.

When the second cancer study was over, a couple of months before we left the old building at Westcott, we were suddenly without any work for our bio-detection dogs, and all of us working on that side of the charity felt low, even though we were busy every day with the diabetes-alert work. Again, it seemed as if the medical profession was determined to ignore the opportunities we were offering it, and late at night I found myself wondering if everything had been in vain. Was I wasting everyone's time pursuing this idea that dogs can detect cancer and save lives? Why were we faced with such a stonewall reaction from the very medical people we wanted to help? It was dispiriting, but deep inside I knew that we were right to keep going, and we tried to not let it get us down.

Our biggest problem, without being involved in a collaborative study, was getting samples for the dogs to train with. We'd lost our supply from Bucks Healthcare NHS Trust. Again, we had a stroke of good luck: we started a collaborative programme with Medical Detection Dogs Italy, an organisation pursuing research on the same lines as ours, and which worked under our aegis. We gave them permission to use the same name. They were happy to provide us with samples, and so our dogs started training on Italian urine samples. We are indebted: without these samples we could not have carried on demonstrating, and that would have seriously affected our ability to raise funds.

We also put out pleas for samples on Facebook and on our own website: 'If you have sadly just been diagnosed with prostate, bladder or kidney cancer, would you consider giving us a urine sample?' We had a host of replies, but most were from people already on treatment. We did find some we could use, and also some good controls: people who had a cancer scare but who had been cleared. Like all our other sample donors, those people made a considerable contribution to getting us through that dark time to where we are now.

We never stopped training the bio-detection dogs, and we started holding more open days to raise our profile. For me and the team it is an everyday thing, watching a dog unerringly sniff out a cancer sample. But people who have never seen it before often have tears in their eyes as they watch the dogs, working for nothing more than a treat or a couple of minutes' play chasing a ball. In the early days we held open days every six to eight weeks, with perhaps ten people at each. But by 2012 we were holding them every four weeks, with thirty or forty people coming each time. The dogs know they have an audience, but it does not put them off: in fact, they seem to appreciate the odd round of applause!

Thankfully, the training of medical alert dogs continued to grow, and we soon needed more space. I was disappointed when another tenant moved into one of the other units, but luckily for us they did not stay long and we were able to take it over. We had a long-term rental agreement for the middle section, but for this other unit we could only have a short-term let, so we negotiated to buy it, with a mortgage. By this time we had changed the name of the charity: in August 2011, we ceased to be Cancer Bio Detection Dogs and adopted the name Medical Detection Dogs, which we all felt covered the range of our work better.

Then we got some news that really cheered up me and the other bio-detection staff. Royal Canin, the dog-food manufacturers who have always been so generous in their support of us, agreed to sponsor a standalone project to work out just how good a dog's sense of smell is, as well as other aspects of their olfaction. We did not need to wait for cancer samples because we were investigating how low a threshold the dogs could reach recognising the odour of amyl acetate (it smells a bit like bananas), as well as investigating other aspects of how the dogs signal their decisions.

To simplify it: the best dogs can smell amyl acetate when it is diluted to one in a trillion parts, which is like finding a teaspoonful of sugar in two Olympic swimming pools. The human nose, by contrast, can't function much above one in a thousand.

We looked at whether all dogs operated at the same level, and whether the environment affected the level of a dog's work. We also wanted to know whether, when a dog makes a mistake with odour detection, it is a genuine mistake or a simple throwaway dismissal of the sample, meaning that the dog was unsure whether the odour was there or not. I was particularly interested in this part of the work, as I believe the odour of cancer in urine is quite weak, and we are asking dogs to operate at those levels. I wanted to know: what does a dog do when the task becomes difficult? Can it tell us in some way that it is unsure, or does it simply dismiss the odour and react as if it is definitely not there?

It was an invaluable study, as we were able to adopt a world-first training system that enables the dogs to work as problem-solvers at a higher level. All traditional scent training rewards a dog when it finds what it is looking for. For example, when a drugs-detection dog goes in to help search a house, it gets a reward in the room where it finds drugs. In another room, where there are no drugs, it gets no reward. But I believe that the dog has worked just as hard to ascertain that the room is clear as it did in the room where it found the drugs.

In our cancer work we already trained dogs in a back-to-front way: drugs and explosive dogs start with the smell of the target, but we had to teach dogs to find an ingredient that we cannot isolate ourselves. Now we knew that we should reward the dogs when they told us the ingredient was not there, as well as when it was there. My favourite metaphor for how we train our dogs is to tell people to imagine that we want them to find red flowers in a Monet painting, but they don't know what they are looking for. They can get there by a process of elimination: it's not the colour red we are looking for, it's a red flower. The flowers themselves may be different varieties, some with smaller petals, some with fewer petals, but the common factor is that they are red flowers. The person has to ignore everything else and just tell us when they find a red flower, but equally, they have got to be able to say, with conviction, that in a particular painting there are no red flowers.

So it is with the odour: the dog has to recognise it even if it is not always quite the same, and the dog also has to be able to say when it is not there. The dog is the problem-solver, not us. This is why I believe that dogs are so far ahead of all attempts to build electronic noses: the man-made nose can only recognise exactly what it is programmed to detect, not a pattern that means the same substance is there, albeit slightly different.

Having trained back to front anyway, which was a major breakthrough and flew in the face of what senior people in the world of dog training told me could be done, we were now able to take it a step further, and train for negative results as well as positive ones.

Soon after we reached these conclusions I had another of my serendipitous encounters. I was in Spain giving a paper at a conference on canine training, and sitting at dinner one evening I found myself talking to one of the other participants, Dr Aubrey Fine, a psychologist from California State Polytechnic University. Aubrey specialises in treating children with ADHD, developmental disorders and learning difficulties in parent–child relationships. He is also a highly regarded world expert on the use of animals in therapy.

I explained to him my challenge: the dogs were working their socks off, and were not rewarded when they did not find the odour. To work effectively clinically, I believed it was as important that our dogs told us when cancer was not present as when it was. Aubrey understands the psychology of how dogs work and learn, and he gave me a few suggestions of behaviours we should be looking for. I came home inspired, having met someone who didn't think I was mad, and didn't think we had to stay within the original parameters set up by the scientific studies.

From then on we changed our reward system, looking at the dog not as a machine but as a sensitive biological system, and we started to manipulate the reward system to increase its sensitivity. By rewarding only for positives, we were increasing the risk of false positives – the dog hazarding a guess when it was not sure, in the hope of getting a reward. Now the dog can tell us what it finds without bias. We changed our emphasis from positive finds to correct answers. Occasionally we want to manipulate in favour of more negatives, because we want the dogs to be 100 per cent sure that the cancer odour is there before they give us a positive, at other times we go the other way in order to know if there's just the slightest chance it is there.

It now sounds so obvious, and I found myself thinking: why was I ever doing it the other way? It reminded me of my philosophy course at university: I had come through the woods into the clearing, where everything suddenly seems blindingly straightforward.

This was the main benefit of the Royal Canin amyl acetate study, but we learned other things too. Some dogs could smell the dilute compound at much lower levels than others, and that may because of their inherent personality, and their ability to focus and concentrate more, but we need to understand this better. We already know that some breeds are better than others: clearly, dogs like pugs have been bred to have their olfactory organs squashed, whereas Labradors and spaniels have had theirs honed over generations. (Pugs have only 250 million odour receptors, compared to 300 million for Labradors.) But we want to know why one Labrador is better than another Labrador. Do they simply have more sensory receptors, or is it to do with the learning process? If we tested two siblings who look identical, we found that right down at the olfactory threshold they differed.

What we need to learn now is what mixture of things makes one dog fantastic, like Dill, Tangle or Daisy, and another average, and we need to devise a way of picking out the experts. We have seen that inexperienced dogs work more quickly than the experienced ones, who take their time, as if to say that they know what they are doing is difficult, and should be given due consideration. I have also observed personally that when I work with a dog I don't particularly like (there are a few ...) and the dog senses this and doesn't like me, it will still work, but to a much lower level than when it is paired with a trainer it likes. It is always a symbiotic relationship, and dogs are so good at reading our feelings that we cannot pretend to them. Dogs are, in fact, the only other animal apart from humans who automatically gaze leftwards when they look at a person, because it is the right-hand side of the human face that most clearly expresses emotions. After centuries of evolution, dogs can read us as well as we read each other.

My lovely Dill was a professor of dogs – but why? Was it because of his incredible breeding from top working dogs? Was it the way I brought him up and developed his brain when he was tiny? Was it rewards? Or was his olfactory system simply better?

We've bred this amazing animal, the dog, and we've restricted it by training it in the ways that suit us, not the ways that suit the dog and bring out the best in him. We are only scratching the surface, there is so much more to learn.

One aspect of the Royal Canin amyl acetate study was published in 2014, written up by a Lincoln University PhD student, Astrid Concha. She recorded whether there was a difference in the way the dogs behaved when they reacted positively or negatively to a sample. Slowed down on film, there is a difference, whereas to the handler it is imperceptible. When the dog sniffs a true negative sample, he spends about half the time sniffing than when it is a positive sample, and this shows up in the slow-motion video. It's exciting because it means the dog's spontaneous behavious is identifying the positive samples, even before he uses the signals we have taught him, to sit and lie down. Again, this made me aware of how much more dogs have to communicate, how much of the information they give us we have yet to decode.

Doing a research programme with something as easily obtainable as amyl acetate was important because it means we have something tangible we can use to compare our dogs with the electronic noses that are being developed. We are able to say: bring your electronic noses and let's see if they can match what our dogs can do. In fact, some time later, that's exactly what happened. One of the noses, which worked well detecting explosives, took part in the comparison. The results are illuminating. Our dogs spend about a second detecting amyl acetate in sample dilutions down to one in a trillion, whereas the electronic nose bottoms out at one part per 50 million, and take fifteen minutes per sample.

This doesn't negate the effectiveness of the nose in finding explosives, but explosives usually come in substantial amounts, enough to make a bomb or other device, so the scent signal is strong. Cancer odours are so much more elusive.

After the Royal Canin study, I retired Tangle from bio-detection work. He was ten and a half, and although he was still working at a very high level, he was showing signs of slowing down a bit in his play, and I felt he deserved a bit more time to sleep and relax.

At about this time I took on another dog of my own, Midas. I had only been living with two dogs since Woody's death, the smallest number for many years. As is the way of things, Midas came into my life and I couldn't say no to her. Again, although I love chocolate-brown cocker spaniels, I didn't want a dog I would be comparing to Dill and Woody, however much I tried not to. With hindsight, I can see I did not want to be reminded of my old life, my marriage years.

Midas is a wire-haired Hungarian vizsla, a relatively rare breed originally bred for hunting. Vizslas have a good sense of smell, intelligence, trainability and affectionate natures, which makes Midas in many ways the perfect bio-detection dog. In common with other vizslas, she's a very lively dog.

Midas arrived when one of our staff had a bitch who had a litter of puppies, all of which were sold. But the new owners of Midas returned her very quickly, unable to keep her as one of their children proved to be allergic to dogs. I said I would adopt her: she was a new breed to me, and it would be a challenge. It certainly has been. Midas matured late, and it was only when she was about three years old that she began to calm down, when we could clearly see her potential in the bio-detection room. It has taken longer for me to train her than it did with Tangle and Daisy. Her protective streak is well developed, and she has an instinct to guard me, which I have to curb – although when I arrive home on a dark evening and take the dogs out for a walk, I always feel secure with Midas.

I chose her name for the same reason as her breed: I didn't want to continue my tradition of Thomas Hardy names, I wanted something different. Midas is the king who in Greek mythology turns everything he touches to gold, and as the dog is a russet/gold colour, it seemed appropriate. I think I also hoped she would bring some of the fortune to us that her namesake generated, and she has been lucky for us, helping with lots of publicity work because she is very photogenic, with her distinguished bearing and slightly patrician air.

She is an interesting dog, and I have learned from her. She is not another soul mate for me: she fits more into

Minstrel's mode, a dog who teaches me a great deal in terms of refining and perfecting my training techniques. But she's more trainable than the eccentric Minstrel was, and I am fascinated by the way she communicates. I have not taught her to do this, but if she wants something she sits and stares at it, without wavering, perhaps giving a little whine. If, after some minutes, I fail to respond, she will put a paw on my knee and then turn and look at the object she wants. Is this instinctive behaviour, or has she learned it? I believe she has worked it out for herself.

My story is punctuated by moments of great good fortune. For all the sticks I have been hit with (according to the teller) and all the problems I have faced, there have been an equal number of times when providence has offered me a road to go down, or brought a person into my life, which has led on to greater things for the work I do. There are so many junctures when I could have followed a different route, but by instinct more than by calculated decision, I always chose the way that would lead on to this ultimate goal: the use and acceptance of the great gift that dogs offer to mankind. There was no grand plan, but when I look back I can see that everything I did, from childhood onwards, pointed me in this direction.

As for the people, there, too, I have been tremendously fortunate. Which brings me to another, very special, supporter who has helped to increase our public profile exponentially. It could so nearly not have happened . . .

Betsy Duncan Smith is the wife of Iain Duncan Smith, the former cabinet minister and one-time leader of the Conservative Party. Her involvement with us has opened many doors, yet again it was serendipity that brought us together.

Betsy was diagnosed with breast cancer in 2009, and unfortunately hers was a much more serious and advanced case than mine. She had chemotherapy, to which she reacted badly, and she was very ill for many months. She had several emergency admissions to hospital, more operations, and spent a gruelling two years recovering. So when in 2012 a friend suggested that she come along to one of our open days, when the dogs demonstrate what they can do and I talk about our work, she was reluctant.

In her words: 'My life had been dominated by cancer for so long, I wanted to get away from it. But my friend knows I am a doggie person, and she insisted I go with her. Like everyone who sees the dogs working, I was amazed and very moved.'

She echoed what Lesley Nicol said: 'It seemed to me so blindingly obvious that dogs can do this: why on earth has it not been harnessed before?'

Betsy immediately said she would help with fundraising, and it was decided to ask her if she would agree to become one of our trustees, as she has lots of good contacts and I hoped she could open doors for us. Although we were getting more and more support, there was still a very stubborn resistance from the medical establishment.

'I didn't think I had any useful contacts,' Betsy said, 'but I was so fired up by what I had seen that whoever I was sitting next to at a lunch or a dinner was told all about the wonderful work going on at MDD.'

Betsy invited Stephan Shakespeare, the founder of the opinion poll company YouGov, and his wife to a fund-raiser for Medical Detection Dogs, which was held on a riverboat on the Thames. The following day, Stephan rang Betsy to say he had carried out an unofficial poll asking ordinary people: 'Would you be happy for dogs to be used in medical diagnosis?' The answer was a resounding 78 per cent in favour, which confirmed our view that the public supported our work.

Soon after we met, Betsy made a pivotal suggestion. She proposed that we write to Camilla, Duchess of Cornwall, and invite her to come to see our work at MDD. I was floored: it would never have occurred to me to presume that a senior member of the royal family would be interested in what we were doing. But Betsy pointed out that both the Duchess and her husband Prince Charles are very fond of dogs, and they are also interested in different ways of expanding medical knowledge and research.

'I think the Duchess will be fascinated by what you are doing here,' she said to me.

Betsy knew one of the Duchess's private secretaries, Jonathan Hellewell, who had previously worked for her husband Iain, so she emailed him. I thought: nothing ventured, nothing gained. Jonathan suggested Betsy meet Amanda MacManus and Joy Camm, assistant private secretaries to Prince Charles and the Duchess, at Clarence House. Betsy knew immediately on meeting them that they 'got' what it is about – in fact, they had clearly researched our work before she arrived. They said they felt the Prince of Wales and the Duchess would be interested in our charity, and after meeting Betsy both Joy and Amanda came to visit us. They were really taken with watching the dogs at work, and at their suggestion we decided to write and invite the Duchess.

The letter went off, and I was expecting that we would have to wait at least twelve months for a visit, as there must be a lot of pressure on the Duchess's diary. Just before the Christmas break in 2012 we received a reply, saying the Duchess would be very interested in coming, and that we would receive a date for the visit soon.

I was astonished when I opened my mail on the first day back in the office after the break to find a letter saying the Duchess was looking forward to coming on 20 February. Wow! We were going to have a royal visit! Everyone was so excited, but suddenly there were only about seven weeks to organise everything. The first problem was space. We wanted to invite our trustees, and some of our clients with medical alert dogs, and whenever there is a royal visit the dignitaries from the county come, and to maximise publicity we needed to invite the press. How on earth were we going to get everyone in?

Dad came to the rescue again. Our neighbours in the unit on the other side of us had recently moved out. They had used the unit for storage of aircraft engines, so it was oily and filthy, but at least it was empty. Dad negotiated with them and discovered that they owned the unit, and were willing to rent it to us. Like all these things, it took a few weeks to finalise, and we actually got the keys a week before the big day.

The state of it was daunting, but my boyfriend Rob got stuck in, working incredibly long hours, snatching just three or four hours' sleep some nights, scrubbing the filthy walls, putting coat after coat of white paint over them, ripping up the oily carpet tiles, getting rid of the engine debris, and fitting the lovely red carpet tiles that one of our supporters donated to us. The carpet tiles run through the other two sections of our building, and there were enough left in storage for Rob to finish the third unit.

Rob Harris worked as Rob's labourer, running around fetching and carrying, and anyone else who was free lent a hand. The work was finally finished at midnight on the night before the visit, and none of us will forget how hard Rob worked to get us there. There were a few of us lending a hand that evening: me, Rob Harris, Simone and anyone else on the staff who was happy to give up their time. There's a joke that the royal family think the world smells of fresh paint because everywhere they go on official visits, someone has spruced the place up. Well, ours was a very big spruce . . .

When Rob finished, we had a large empty space that was not linked internally to the rest of our building, but it gave us somewhere to allow all our guests in. We needed a barrier to keep most of our guests – and their dogs – back, to allow the Duchess to move along and meet them. Mum and Dad generously sourced, paid for and donated to us a queue control barrier, with stainless steel posts and red retractable belts between them. On the morning of the visit, sixty people – trustees, supporters, volunteers and clients with their dogs – filled the empty space.

That morning I washed my hair and dressed in the new suit that Mum and Dad had insisted I buy. Mum said: 'Claire, we're not leaving this to chance,' and they dragged me off round the shops like a reluctant teenager, thrusting different outfits into my hand and pushing me into dressing rooms. The suit we chose has a long black skirt and a jacket, also black, but softened with a slight white fleck. When I got to the office, my hair was styled by Lydia Swanson, one of our dog trainers, who has volunteered as my chief hairdresser, as she can be relied upon to make me look presentable whenever television cameras – or royal visitors – appear.

Rob Harris and I were in the large demo room, checking we had the right urine samples to be used on the carousel, when a shout went up: 'Claire, Claire! She's here!' I was still wearing plastic gloves to handle the samples.

I suppose I assumed a royal visit might start a few minutes late – after all, I'm famously last-minute, as everyone will tell you. But the Duchess arrived slightly early. I tore through the building, ripping the gloves off and throwing them to one side, to reach the front door in the nick of time. The dignitaries were lined up and being introduced by the Lord Lieutenant of the county when I managed to get myself on to the end of the line, just in time.

Then I escorted the Duchess into the building, introducing John Church, without whom none of this would have happened, and the medics who had already come on board to support us, including the eminent oncologist Professor Karol Sikora, diabetes specialist Dr Vicky Horden, medical advisor Dr Carol Tang and oncologist Dr Alan Makepeace. All our trustees, including Betsy and her husband Iain, and our ambassador Lesley Nicol, were there.

Next I introduced her to the staff training medical alert dogs. The first in line went well: the trainer was holding the puppy who was being trained as the first dog in the world to alert a client with POTS. The puppy, called Charlie, received a royal stroke. But the next trainer shouted 'Hello', then performed a strange curtsey. Next in line was my sister Simone, who got the curtsey right but dried up completely when the Duchess asked: 'How did you hear about the charity?'

Simone stared at her blankly, as if she were talking a foreign language. The Duchess moved along the line and the next trainer, Kimberly, blurted out, 'I'm a Type 1 diabetic,' before the Duchess had a chance to speak. The Duchess told Kimberly that she was a patron of a charity for young diabetics, and Kimberly blurted out again, 'I'm a Type 1 diabetic.'

I found it hard to suppress a giggle at the way my competent, bright, hard-working, eminently sensible staff had become incoherent, babbling idiots. The Duchess must get it all the time, because she kept a straight face and was charming to everyone.

Betsy was right: the Duchess did find the work fascinating. She watched Rob Harris work Daisy round the carousel, unerringly identifying the samples with cancer. Then she watched a very young diabetes-alert dog, Pippin, demonstrate how she reacts to clicker training, learning to alert. Like so many others who actually see these enthusiastic animals at work, her eyes misted up.

After the demonstration I took her outside to walk round to the big, new room where so many more people, and dogs, were waiting to greet her. I explained to her that we had only just acquired the building, and would be knocking it through to the rest of the building as soon as we could. One of our young clients, Alena, was waiting with her diabetes-alert dog Maisie to present a posy of roses and daffodils.

At the end of her visit the Duchess unveiled a plaque. Instead of the usual red curtain covering it, we used one of our special MDD red dog coats. The Duchess said a few words: 'I am incredibly impressed and staggered by the work that is done here. You can read about these things but you have to be able to see it to believe it. More people should know about it, congratulations to you all.'

As she left, the Duchess quietly said to me: 'I'm going to tell my husband about you.'

The royal visit gave us an enormous boost because pictures of the event appeared in national as well as local newspapers, and I was inundated with requests to give talks. But the royal support didn't end there. A few months later, Betsy and I were invited to meet Mark Leishman, private secretary to Prince Charles and the Duchess of Cornwall.

'The Prince is very interested in your work. Can you tell me about it?' he said.

I spoke for about two minutes, outlining what we do as briefly as I could. Mark listened attentively, then said: 'How can we help? Would you like a reception at Highgrove? Or an event at Clarence House?'

I nearly fell off my chair, and Betsy looked just as amazed. I think we sat there for a few seconds with our mouths open like goldfish. In the end it was clear that an event at Clarence House would be the best option. It was an amazing and completely unexpected moment, and I struggle to find words to say what a fantastic feeling it was. We had hit so many brick walls trying to convince people of the importance of the work, and now the Prince of Wales and Duchess of Cornwall were throwing their weight behind us.

The invitations were sent out in the name of the Prince of Wales himself – a great honour, as we were expecting to send them out ourselves and put 'in the presence of HRH Prince Charles and the Duchess of Cornwall'. Receiving invitations direct from the Prince more or less guaranteed that all the top doctors and scientists working in cancer detection and representatives of other cancer charities agreed to come. The Prince's staff and I worked out a joint list. Many of the guests had been invited before to come to see our work, but only a few had made their way to Milton Keynes to meet us. But a summons from the Prince of Wales proved much more effective in drumming up support. Before the big day, the venue was changed to the magnificent throne room at St James's Palace, to accommodate everyone and to make sure there was room for our carousel.

It was during the preparation for the event that, at Betsy's suggestion, I plucked up the courage to discuss with her aides if it would be appropriate to ask the Duchess if she would consider being the patron of MDD. I knew it would be a while before I found out if she had agreed: palace staff had to check out the bona fides of the charity, and I fully understand how they have to be sure about us. I heard, unofficially, that we came out very well in the checks, especially for our meticulous evidence-based science. I also know that we have relatively small administrative costs compared to many charities, and that, because of this, a bigger percentage of our money goes into training our assistance dogs. But it was a nail-biting time waiting to hear if MDD would make the grade.

In the meantime, though, I had much to think about. In the run-up to the event, everyone was asking me if I had prepared my speech. I never do normally, but I wondered whether I should at least have notecards and bullet points to remind me what I needed to get across. People said: 'How will you know exactly how long you have been talking without a speech?'

I knew my timing had to be spot on because Charles and Camilla work on a very tight timetable, and I also knew that this was the biggest opportunity I had ever had to impress the people who really needed to know about us, the medical profession and the scientists. I worried over it, and then, a couple of days before the event, I woke in the middle of the night with a clear conviction that I should do it the way I always do, speaking from somewhere deep inside me. I never know where it comes from, but I now give so many talks and presentations that when I open my mouth the story of the dogs and our work with them just flows. I never write it down.

The day before the event we heard some momentous news: one of the Duchess's aides rang to say that she had agreed to be our patron. A letter of confirmation arrived a couple of days later. It was a wonderful boost to my confidence.

The night before the big event I was awake until 3am, desperately trying to get some footage of our work over to the BBC, who wanted to do an item on us to coincide with our visit to St James's Palace. For some reason that is completely beyond me, their computer and my computer were not on speaking terms, and it was a struggle trying different ways to get the film across.

I remember thinking: this is going to be one of the biggest days in my life, and I am still up at 3am the night before, and everyone thinks I should have written a speech but I haven't . . . I slipped into the meditation mode that I learned in Korea, and told myself: 'This is not about you, Claire Guest; it's about dogs and what they can do for us. You have less than half an hour to engage everyone who is there. Forget everything else; forget your ego. This is the biggest opportunity of your life to expound the cause. Focus on the dogs.'

It was a very early start for Simone and our patron Lesley Nicol, as they had to be at the studio of the ITV *Daybreak* programme by 6am, taking Patmore, the poodle named after Lesley's character in *Downton*. Then they made a mad dash through the traffic to arrive on time at the palace, where they were met at the door by royal aides. Simone knew that Patmore needed a toilet break, and was expecting to take her to St James's Park. But she was assured it was all right to go into the palace gardens, and she was shown the way.

We learned later that the Duchess looked out of a window, spotted Patmore about her business, and said to Prince Charles: 'Someone's walking their dog in the garden.'

Luckily an aide was on hand to explain it was one of our dogs. They both thought it was hilarious. When we chatted about it later the Duchess said she didn't associate our dogs with poodles, so it was a surprise. I'm pleased to say that Simone had a poo bag with her: we didn't leave any souvenirs in the royal garden.

The throne room is splendid, with rich red carpet, gilt decorations, huge portraits on the wall, glistening chandeliers and, at one end, the canopied throne surrounded by deep red velvet drapes. I had no time to absorb the great sense of history that pervades such a special place: I had to make sure the carousel was working, and that all our clients with their dogs were happy. Betsy was worried that one of the dogs would cock its leg over something priceless, but I had given everyone who brought a dog instructions to make sure they had a good long toilet break before coming inside.

I gave my talk, and it was exactly the right length, twenty-two minutes. Afterwards, someone said to me, 'You must have practised that for weeks.' He could hardly believe it when I said I had spoken off the cuff. But I knew every aspect of what I wanted to say, and I didn't miss any of the important points. Although I never write my talks, I do tailor them to the audience: more about science and medicine if I am talking to scientists and doctors, more about the human stories when I am helping to raise funds.

We had never dismantled the carousel and taken it out of the training centre before but, as ever, when the dogs worked round it their ability to alert meant so much more than any number of words. Three dogs were used, and the room fell silent as everyone watched them start sniffing round the plates, always alerting at the cancer sample. Lucy sniffed out bladder cancer. Daisy, who had by this time screened more than 6,000 samples with a 93 per cent success rate, was given the difficult task of finding a very early stage renal cancer. Finally, Ulric easily found the prostate cancer sample. There were gasps each time, as the dogs got it right, and I could see the body language of some of the most hardened sceptics begin to change. The comedian Bill Bailey, who is an ambassador for a prostate cancer char-ity, and who had been working to raise awareness of the disease, had tears in his eyes.

'Both the Duchess and I had an emotional reaction, and I wasn't expecting that,' he said to me later. 'I was expecting a clinical trial. It brought a lump to my throat and a tear to my eye. How many lives could this save?'

After me, there was a talk from Claire Pesterfield who is one of our clients with diabetes. Claire is much more than a client: she is a very good speaker, who can con-vey what it is like to have the full-time help of her dog, Magic, far better than I can. She is a paediatric diabetes nurse, and says that when her own diabetic highs and lows became hard to detect and she was collapsing and becoming very ill, the paramedics who loaded her into their ambulances would look askance when she told them what her job is.

'They seemed to think that I, of all people, should be handling my diabetes better. But I had ceased to have any awareness of my blood sugars falling or rising,' she said in her speech.

Magic, a yellow Labrador, who Claire describes as 'a clumsy muppet', has the awareness she lacks, and thrusts her kit at her whenever he scents her levels changing, giving her as much as a forty-minute warning.

'Life has changed beyond measure since Magic came into my life. My husband, my parents, everyone who cares about me, can now relax, knowing I am in very good hands,' she said. Claire has worked for us on a research project into the enhanced quality of life our diabetic clients have, and the cost-effectiveness of assistance dogs. She talks so well, I want to let her say, in her own words, what she has now told many distinguished gatherings. I can't better her words:

Imagine life with an incurable disease that impacts every minute of every day of your life. Imagine a relentless battle for health, struggling every day to keep a balance, pretending that you are normal and can carry on.

Imagine being reliant on others to participate in everyday activities like going to the cinema, shopping or going to work. Imagine being afraid to go to sleep for fear of never waking up. Imagine the exhaustion of waking every hour, night after night, in the hope that you will prevent the episode that may otherwise kill you.

Many people don't have to imagine. They have this existence day after day. They wonder what the future may hold, many not daring to plan ahead for fear that today may be their last. Partners, parents, children and friends continually worry about what they may come home to.

Now imagine a four-legged friend, his devotion only bettered by his love of dog biscuits, bacon, cheese whirlers and a tummy tickle. Imagine a dog jumping on your bed at 3 am, warning you to take action now, before it is too late. Imagine a dog saving your life, day after day, night after night. For me, that dog is called Magic . . . I owe my life to Medical Detection Dogs. I now not only imagine what my life could be like, I now live it.

After Claire's moving talk, it was time for the Duchess and the Prince of Wales to mingle with our guests, the Duchess crouching down on the floor to talk to Cerys Davies and her dog Wendy. They chatted to Lesley, our ambassador, and also to Yasmine Torblad, whose black poodle, Nano, was the first nut-allergy dog to be trained in Europe.

Prince Charles talked to me and told me he was very impressed by the way we were making sure that all our work was scientifically monitored and evidence-based. He said it is also important not to restrict ourselves and close our minds to what is available to us.

So many people came up to me to say that they had not believed in our work until that day. They had doubted us, and ignored previous invitations to see us. Now they were even offering help to obtain samples. For the first time, I felt that the doctors and scientists talked to me as an equal, and treated me, not just as a crank with a theory on the wilder shores of medical research, but as someone with a real knowledge and skill that could change lives.

After the demonstration, tea was served in the Queen Mother's drawing room. Aides were reminding Prince Charles and the Duchess that it was time for them to leave for another engagement, and I walked downstairs with them, both of them talking enthusiastically about our work. As we approached the main door of the palace, Simone came back in, having once again been attending to Patmore's needs. She spotted me and shouted 'Hi!' breezily, only then glancing at my companions ...

Having royal patronage is amazing and definitely affects the way we are viewed by the public in general. For me it is a huge thing: there have been times when I have felt almost overwhelmed by the tidal wave of scepticism that we have ridden since the very early days. At last, we were coming clear of all the disbelief and dismissal.

I've realised that there are two distinct cynical attitudes to our work. The diehards are those who say that dogs can never help medically, and just because we prove that dogs can do it, nonetheless it will never be of any practical use, so let's forget it. The second group are not so much sceptics as people who believe in it, but are sceptical about our approach to it, not accepting the need to use it in a harnessed, scientific way. They say: 'Why don't you just get on and do it? People will pay to have their urine screened. What are you waiting for? You could be saving lives right now. It's wrong to delay . . .'

Of course, that would be a totally unregulated service open to all sorts of abuse. The only way forward is evidence-based work, but never disregarding the fact that the dog is a biological system and not a machine, and needs and offers companionship alongside this amazing ability.

I was very pleased that among our medical guests on that momentous day was Dr Iqbal Anjum, a consultant urologist working at Milton Keynes University Hospital. His support has proved invaluable to us, and it is with him that we have embarked on a three-year clinical trial that will culminate in dogs actually being used as part of the diagnostic process for bladder, prostate and kidney cancer patients.

This is the way forward.

CHAPTER TWELVE

Sylvia

'Would you like to tell us about your work? As executors of a will, we have some funds to allocate to charity, and we're interested to hear about your work and what you would do with any money we might allocate to you.'

The letter came completely out of the blue. It was an unusual request, but I was obviously very happy to send information. Then came a reply, inviting me to travel to the solicitors' offices in London to talk to the executors in person. All I was told was that a lady had died and left instructions for the bulk of her estate to go to charity, but she had not stipulated which charities, although she had left some guidelines. She was interested in animals, but did not necessarily want to leave the money to an animal charity: she was more concerned with it going to organisations that helped with unusual health conditions.

I was not the only charity boss invited to give a presentation. I had no idea how much money was involved, but I felt it must be at least £5,000 for them to be going to the lengths of interviewing people. I was asked to tell the executors what we would do with an injection of money into Medical Detection Dogs.

It was a little bit unnerving, walking into a room and talking to a small panel of people, two men and one woman. It reminded me of the television programme, *Dragons' Den*. By this time I had given many talks and interviews, but even so I felt I needed moral support, so Betsy Duncan Smith came with me. I decided not to be nervous: I had no idea what the stakes were, so I was not going to worry about them if I could help it.

I told the executors that one of our most pressing needs was the funding for another trainer in our assistance dog work. I showed some videos, including those of our clients who have dogs, explaining the impact on their lives that the dogs have made. I also talked about our cancer work, and how vital it was to get beyond the testing stage and to be able to bring it in to practical use to help save lives.

But I decided to pitch really high, share my dream with them. Dad had prepared plans for me, showing the buildings we work in, and the land around them, and I explained that in a perfect world it would be wonderful to own them, to give the charity a secure base, and eventually to perhaps have a new building on the site.

I left feeling I had given them a good taste of our work, but I knew that other charities were pitching, so I was not confident we would get any money. I put the episode out of my mind.

A couple of weeks later, I had a phone call from the solicitor who had chaired the panel of executors. Yes, we had received an award from the will.

Eight hundred thousand pounds.

I have no words to sum up how I felt when I heard the figure. I had to ask her to repeat it. Eight hundred thousand. Wow! I had no clue it would be such a large amount. There have been many turning points, vital moments in the history of Medical Detection Dogs, but this was a big one. I rang the chairman, Michael Brander, and Dad because he had helped prepare the pitch, but I said nothing to the staff until the letter, confirming the money, landed on my desk. Until I saw it in black and white it did not seem real. As soon as it was official, we cracked open two or three bottles of fizz that I brought in, to celebrate.

I now know a certain amount of information about our benefactor, which the executors have kindly supplied to us. She was a very private person, and I know her only by her first name, Sylvia. She lived with her parents, and then on her own, in the family home in Buckinghamshire. Her paternal grandparents were German, and her mother escaped from Austria just before the Second World War. Sylvia's family felt this country had been good to them, and she wanted to give something back.

She loved her family home, which had beautiful gardens. Sadly, she suffered from ill health for much of her life, including having anorexia when she was a teenager, which had a long-term detrimental effect on her health. When she was well enough, she worked as a medical secretary, and from that stemmed her interest in medical developments.

Her father died unexpectedly from a heart attack, and her mother died a few years before Sylvia, at a time when Sylvia was also critically ill. After her mother's death, she fought hard to preserve her independence and dignity, living at home with live-in carers. It was important to her that people should have the choice to die where they wanted and with the support they needed and deserved.

She loved children and young people and understood they need special treatment and the right environment when they are ill.

The executors said that Sylvia would have been delighted to help Medical Detection Dogs with securing premises for the future, training more dogs, and supporting the studies into prostate and breast cancer detection.

I know we were not the only charity to receive a substantial donation, and it is very hard to put into words how I feel about her, a woman who was clearly much loved in life and who, in death, allowed us, and others, to move forward with our work. When I think about her I feel quite emotional and sad that she will never know how much good she has done, and that she was never able to come here and see what we do. The executors of her will, who speak very fondly of her, have since been here and seen the dogs working, and been shown what we have been able to do with her money.

With this huge amount in our bank, we were able to buy all three units of the building, paying off the mortgage on one and buying the other two, plus the paddock and a field and small copse adjacent to the building.

Some of the money funded our getting through protocol and ethics for a third study into cancer detection, which meant training Daisy and Lucy to see if they could detect more than one cancer from urine, starting with bladder and prostate. (This study was later subsumed into the big, three-year trial we are currently carrying out with Milton Keynes Hospital.) More went into the training of our medical alert dogs, and everything else was used as a deposit on the new buildings that we are putting up to enable us to have more than one bio-detection room operating. With more than twenty-five dogs now trained or in training for the cancer-detection work, the only things that limit us are the constant need for more samples, and having only one room to work the dogs in.

The third unit of the building, the one that we acquired immediately before the Duchess of Cornwall visited, was kitted out to a very high standard by a generous grant from the Wolfson Foundation, a charitable organisation founded by the Wolfson family, and which by the time it reached its sixtieth anniversary in 2015 had donated £1.7 billion in real terms to worthy causes. One of the original aims of the foundation is to support medical research, and that's how we were chosen for funding.

The money means the unit now has washable floors, rather than the carpet tiles we hurriedly laid for the royal visit, which were carefully lifted and re-used elsewhere. It is, after all, a controlled environment where the dogs work, and needs to be washed down every day after use. There is a 5 metre by 2.5 metre glass wall, behind which visitors can stand or sit to see the dogs at work. The dogs are completely used to having spectators. An intercom links the working area with the viewing area, so that the trainers can tell the audience exactly what is happening, and where the cancer sample is placed on the carousel. There are audible gasps from visitors when, time after time, the dogs find the right sample.

The bio-detection dogs have their own entrance to the building: not that the office staff don't enjoy seeing them when they arrive for work every day. There's office space for the bio-detection team, and an area for the dogs to relax in, with beds and blankets, as well as the paddock where they romp around, always supervised but free to be their doggy selves.

We use the carousel in training, and we also use a four-stand system, where the dogs find a cancer sample from a selection of four, and a yes/no stand, where the dogs are simply offered one sample and they alert when it contains the smell of cancer. We are testing all three systems to see which is the best and most consistent for our major study with Milton Keynes Hospital.

The most exciting development is a stand that allows the dog to press against a pressure point with his nose if he has found a positive sample, and computer software will read his response, so in theory there is no need for a trainer in the room.

Even better, this computer software, developed by Dr Clara Mancini and her team at the Open University, can read how long it takes the dog to decide to press (a 'yes') or move away (a 'no'). This, importantly, tells us when the dog is equivocal about the sample, and it's a 'maybe'. We're hoping to develop this to the point where we can detect when prostate cancer changes from being a pussycat (many older men have it without any serious side effects) to becoming a tiger, a life-threatening, aggressive cancer. In the story of Medical Detection Dogs, there are so many breakthrough moments, and this, we believe, will be another of them. We want to enhance the communication between us and the dogs. This gives them the chance to say: 'Hey, I'm not sure, either, but there may be something here . . .'

By the time the clinicians at Milton Keynes Hospital start receiving reports from us, the dogs will have assessed 3,000 samples. Every sample will be looked at by two dogs looking for bladder cancer, four dogs for prostate cancer, and two for kidney cancer. The results of the study will give us a definitive answer as to how effective this is, and then we will look into whether our work can be used as a diagnostic tool.

It would be amazing if one day this test could be offered to anyone presenting with concerning symptoms. After all, donating a urine sample is so easy, and so many lives can be saved if these cancers are found early.

Our new buildings will house another two bio-detection rooms, and then we will be able to get more dogs on stream, which is vital with all the work we now have lined up. Our bio-detection dogs start work in earnest when they are about a year old. They are socialised and brought up like normal dogs, and they are introduced to the bio-detection surroundings and they watch older dogs working, to see that it's friendly and fun before they start intensive training. Their foster carers are told not to use certain commands, the ones we use when they are working, but apart from that they live like normal pets.

Interestingly, when they come to work, they know they have a job to do. At home they run around, play, sleep on the sofa, all the things dogs do. But they take work seriously, and are always eager for their turn. For demonstrations they wear red coats, like the assistance dogs, but normally in the medical detection room they don't, and it's clearly not the coat that puts them in work mode. We use spaniels and Labradors mainly – we have slightly more spaniels than Labs, usually bred from lines of field-trial cockers or springers. (We have a wider variety of breeds in the Medical Assistance dogs, and we're now training more small dogs for that work, as some of our clients can't accommodate a large dog in their homes.)

As well as the three-year project on prostate, kidney and bladder cancer that we are doing in co-operation with the Milton Keynes hospital, in 2014 we went through NHS ethics to work on the detection of breast cancer through breath samples, with Bucks Healthcare NHS Trust supplying the samples. More than 50,000 people a year are diagnosed with breast cancer, and 12,000 of them die. Women over fifty are screened with mammograms, but they cannot routinely have these more frequently than every three years because of the radiation dangers, so a simple non-invasive breath test would be a major breakthrough.

The work is proving to be very challenging, and we are trying to find better ways to capture the breath samples, as the signal sometimes seems to be there and sometimes so weak that the dogs miss it. We suspect that the filters we are using are trapping the odour too tightly or not at all, and we are looking at other possibilities. Nobody knows better than I do that dogs can detect breast cancer: we simply have to make sure we can harness the way they are doing it.

Like urine samples, breath samples are non-intrusive, and we get them when women are referred to a breast clinic, and are asked if they would take part in a study by breathing into one of our tubes. The samples are coded, and later on, when the mammograms have been read and subsequent diagnosis carried out, we can match the positive samples.

One of our new projects is on the detection of lung cancer. Seventy per cent of lung cancer sufferers present to their specialist when their cancer has reached Stage 4, and for most of them that means they only have six months left to live. So the Holy Grail is to find a simple test that will pick it up far earlier, when the rates for cure are much higher. One eminent specialist is very keen for us to run a study, to help raise the profile of lung cancer, and to help people understand that it is not a self-inflicted disease caused by smoking, but that non-smokers are victims, too.

It costs £250,000 for each two-year cancer study. It sounds a lot, but in terms of medical research it is a very modest amount. Our research also has a very high success level: a major drugs company trials, on average, 500 different possible treatments before they get one that goes on stream and benefits patients. Each drug takes an average of twelve to twenty-five years to develop, and costs $1.7 billion. It makes our diagnostic work seem very cheap.

We hope, eventually, that we will be able to offer the service to hospitals in the same way that Milton Keynes Hospital may, towards the end of the three-year study, add in the information from the dogs as part of the diagnostic process. The dogs will never be the sole arbiter of whether or not someone has prostate, bladder or kidney cancer, but their information will help the clinician decide whether a patient has to come in for further testing. If this happens it will be a world first: it is the first time ever that dogs have been part of the diagnostic process. But research is research, and we can't pre-empt the results.

One of the criticisms we get from the sceptics is: 'It's a dog, it may have an off day ...'

Of course it may. But it's not about one dog randomly sniffing samples. We work in a meticulous, organised, scientific way.

It is not just cancer that we believe can be detected by dogs. We know from our work with assistance dogs that most diseases have a distinctive odour, and we are happy to be taking part in a study into Parkinson's disease. The hope is that by detecting changes in the levels of sebum, an oily substance found on the skin, early detection of Parkinson's will enable doctors to start treatment earlier and prolong a good quality of life for patients. There is anecdotal evidence that the skin of Parkinson's patients changes, and in the early stages they get 'adolescent skin', oilier and sometimes with spots on their faces and backs. We are taking part in a trial co-ordinated by Manchester University to see if there is a role for dogs in detecting these changes. We plan to train two dogs for the work.

We've also had talks about using dogs to test whether infections are bacterial or viral. Over-prescription of anti-biotics is now a serious problem, with the bugs becoming increasingly resistant to them, and a quick and easy way to tell which chest infections will respond to antibiotic treatment would be a major asset. The drugs are effective against bacterial infections but not viral ones. It's a tricky proposition for us, as the conditions under which we carry out any trials will have to be very stringent. The cancer samples are harmless: if there was an accident with a sample, it would simply be a wasted sample. With infectious samples, there are obvious health risks for humans and dogs, so we are investigating the safest ways to present the samples.

There is so much potential. I am advisor to a project using dogs in a hospital for spinal injuries in Hawaii. Dogs were being taken round the wards to give patients a chance to meet and stroke them, when one of the staff of the Assistance Dogs of Hawaii charity noticed that the dogs were reacting to patients who had urinary tract infections. UTIs are the primary medical concern for patients with spinal injuries, and the main reason for them to be admitted to hospital, as they can spread to the kidney and bloodstream, causing sepsis. The need for a permanent catheter greatly increases the risk of infections, and the lack of feeling means that the patient is often very ill before it is detected.

One of the dogs appeared to be alerting in front of a patient whose sample came back negative, but by the time result came in the patient was in intensive care with a raging infection. Clearly, the dog had found something so early it was not yet evident in the sample.

So now they have done a bio-detection study, and their dogs, like ours, are trained in a side room, sniffing samples. New work, which I am advising on, will in future involve training dogs to live at home with people with spinal injuries and alert to UTIs. I must say, there are worse places to have to visit than Hawaii.

Now the dogs are alerting as the infection begins to strike and treatment can start before a culture is grown in a laboratory. The saving in distress to the patient – and money to the health services – is huge.

One of the questions I get asked is: are we going to start our own breeding programme to ensure we have enough suitable dogs? It's something we think about, and it may happen in the future. Personally, I had a couple of attempts at mating Daisy, my wonder dog, but nothing happened. She was a flirt, but she refused to allow a dog to mate with her, even a very suitable candidate who moved in to live with us for a fortnight. Tests at the vet's were inconclusive, but I decided at that stage to get her spayed, as it cuts down on the risk of mammary cancer. When the vet operated he found she had polycystic ovaries, and could never have had puppies.

I was sad, but by then I had accepted I was not going to breed from her. I went back to Bridget, her breeder, but sadly Daisy's line had gone: there was no longer a bitch with Daisy's genes. However, her brother Skipper was happily siring litters of fox-red Labrador pups and I heard there was a lovely bitch pup available. I drove down to Sussex to see the litter, and I admit that she didn't jump out at me at first sight; I didn't have one of those love-at-first-sight moments I have had with some of my dogs. In fact, there was a prettier puppy in the litter I could have had. But I knew she was the right one for me when someone started drilling outside, and the noise and commotion scattered all the puppies. All except her. She sat there, completely unflappable.

When I got Daisy in 2004, fox reds were comparatively rare, but there are more of them about now, and by breeding for colour they now have a tendency to be slightly nervy: when you breed for one characteristic you may accidentally enhance another. A famous experiment dating back over fifty years in Russia shows how breeding foxes selectively, so that the least aggressive ones were bred, turned them in a matter of three generations into animals recognisable as domestic dogs, going from red foxes to look like black-and-white dogs which barked like dogs and had two seasons for mating per year, unlike one for foxes. This is an extreme example of what happens all the time in genetics, and why we have to be very careful breeding dogs – or other animals – for one characteristic.

So the fact that this little Labrador puppy was so fearless, the most confident in the litter, made me choose her. We need confidence and unflappability here. I decided to call her Florin, keeping to the new gold theme I started with Midas. She matured quickly, unlike Midas, and by one year old she was already working well as a bio-detection dog. She's got her own personality and can be rude, ignoring people who want to be friendly with her. She gives a look that says, 'Whatever . . .'

Florin is incredibly motivated by food, so we've harnessed that in her training. Daisy is quite keen on food, but Midas is indifferent to treats. Like all dogs, they put different values on things: Midas likes to own objects, and she'll growl if other dogs go near her bone. Daisy values being praised and looks mortified if she is ever told off: she always wants to please. It's important for anyone who has a dog that they understand what their dog values and what motivates them, and don't try to apply rules without seeing how they impact on that individual.

It seems odd to me when I look at my little pack of dogs that I have ended up with three ginger bitches: Daisy, Midas and Florin. I've always preferred dogs to bitches, and my favourites are chocolate cocker spaniels. Perhaps one day soon I will be ready to have another cocker, probably when I can breed from Dill's frozen sperm. I like having three: more dogs become difficult, it's harder to give each of them the individual time they need with a busy life like mine. On the other hand, with a larger pack you get to see the interaction of the dogs with each other because they are less fixated on human companionship.

The leader of my pack now is Midas, but it's a very harmonious group. Daisy is a brilliant detection dog, operating at levels above all the others, and now our expert consultant, but she is too placid to be a leader, and Florin is too young. So I have a small pack led by a strange wire-haired vizsla.

Our public profile continues to grow, and we have been lucky to be able to show what we can do to lots of influential people. We would love to have official funding, of course, but we accept that there are many other charities who feel the same. But by demonstrating what we do, and getting it talked about, we hope to bring in more and more donors. The amount of work we can do now is limited by lack of resources, and I'd love to see the day when we can bring the waiting list for assistance dogs right down, as well as being able to carry out many more clinical trials in bio detection.

The help that Betsy and her husband Iain have given to us in opening doors cannot be overestimated. Off the back of our demonstration at St James's Palace we were invited to the House of Lords, again to demonstrate with the carousel. It was a bad day for me, as I had lost my sense of balance through an ear infection, and I was staggering a bit. My GP told me not to go, but I am determined never to lose the opportunity to proselytise about our work. Somehow, adrenalin kicked in, and I managed to give my talk as usual. Afterwards, on the way to find a taxi, I felt really sick and was rolling about like a drunk, and Betsy had to steady me. It was well worth the effort, as Lord Trees, a cross-bench peer and a vet, has become a dedicated supporter of MDD.

I was thrilled and amazed by the interest we were getting. Betsy and I also went to meet John Baron, the chairman of the All Party Parliamentary Group on Cancer, an organisation dedicated to keeping cancer high on the parliamentary agenda. He arranged for us to take a small delegation to their annual conference, and to lay on a demonstration with the dogs. Iain also invited Jeremy Hunt, the Secretary of State for Health, to come on an official visit to our headquarters to see what we do. He commented that it was an amazing place. Later he said: 'I was really impressed with what I saw. Both we and NHS England will look very closely at the outcome of the (Milton Keynes) trial.'

After his visit, Sean Duffy, the National Clinical Director for Cancer for NHS England, came to see us and watched the dogs working. Mr Duffy admitted he was sceptical, but he was converted when he saw how robust the science is behind our work.

Another memorable occasion for me was meeting Mark Harper, when he was Minister for Disabled People. I stayed in London the night before, but managed to get lost and ended up crossing the Thames on the wrong bridge, and having to sprint to Westminster. Thank goodness I keep up my running . . . After the meeting I had to ask one of Iain's aides for some plasters because my feet were bleeding.

Another of our lucky breaks is that our local MP is John Bercow, the Speaker of the House of Commons. He has always been a supporter, and has visited to see our work. As Speaker, he can give a certain number of charity events a year at Speaker's House, in the precincts of the Houses of Parliament. We asked him if it would be possible to hold an event there, and he readily agreed. We invited a mixture of eminent consultants, scientists, donors and MPs. Two of the diabetes dogs which came with us gave their owners a sugar alert while we were there: what better demonstration of how vital they are? Claire Pesterfield, whose dog Magic was one of those that alerted, as usual spoke very movingly. We have been lucky enough to do more demonstrations there.

Some of our dogs have even travelled abroad with us. The International Federation for Animal Health invited us to its annual European Pet Night Event, in Brussels. I went with Daisy, and delivered my usual talk, but it was Gemma Faulkner and her dog Polo who stole the show. We were all very proud and tearful to hear Gemma, who was twelve at the time, talking so confidently about how her life has changed since she has had Polo by her side. As she spoke, Polo seemed to sit up straighter, as if he knew he was being lavished with praise.

Daisy is an experienced traveller. When I took her to Milan to work with our Italian colleagues there was some publicity about her, and she was even pursued along the street by paparazzi. Like all the greatest stars, she turned her beautiful face to the cameras and calmly walked on.

It was a great honour for me to be invited to a Buckingham Palace garden party in May 2015. I took as my guest Anne Mills, who worked then as an administrator and as my PA, and who was brilliant at keeping my hectic life in order. It was my thank you to her for coping with it all: balancing my work as chief executive of the charity with also being head of operations is a triumph of her organisational skills. She's now our fundraising and external donors manager.

For our big date at the palace I raided Mum's wardrobe, not for the first time. Mum is much smaller in height than me, but I have long known that her smart suits fit me: I obviously wear them shorter than she does. The one I chose for that day was a purple suit, which was almost new, and which Mum has now given to me. I teamed it with a large hat I found in a charity shop. Camilla, the Duchess of Cornwall, selected me as one of the people she wanted to talk to, and when her aide started to make the introduction I was amazed that she said: 'I know who Claire is . . .'

A marvellous postscript to our relationship with the Duchess of Cornwall came in early 2015, when her private secretary Amanda phoned to say that, for the first time, the Duchess had decided to sell the honey she produces from beehives in her private garden in Wiltshire. Jars of the honey were available at Fortnum and Mason, at the international Eurostar terminus at St Pancras Station and at Heathrow Terminal Five. It was an honour that, out of all the charities she supports, she chose us to receive all her profits.

We owe so much to Betsy Duncan Smith for help in raising our profile. But Betsy has not simply been concerned with introducing us to influential people. She has also worked very hard engaging the local community in our work. She has contacted local shops, businesses and schools on our behalf, and several local schools have now taken up our cause and raised funds for us. We have had sixth formers who are studying science come to our demonstrations. Betsy and a friend have also set up what is, I think, going to be an annual fundraiser for us: Dogs' Day Out, when working dogs and family pets are invited to take part in fun events and challenges, while spectators enjoy a barbecue, country stalls, tractor rides and fun competitions.

We've added three more ambassadors to join Lesley Nicol: we now have Kate Humble, the television presenter best known for her wildlife programmes, Gillian Wright, the actress who is in *EastEnders*, and Debbie Flint, author and QVC presenter. They have supported our stand at Crufts, and done many other charity events for us. It's amazing the difference a celebrity can make in attracting people to our stand.

But although celebrities help, I never lose sight of the people who collect for us at all sorts of events up and down the country, some of them attending fêtes and fairs in all weathers, and our clients who proudly take their dogs, in their red coats, with them on sponsored walks and to community events to let people know about the work we do. Without our volunteers and fundraisers, we would be lost.

The Royal Canin study helped raise awareness of our work in the scientific community. I was already being targeted for advice by dog-training facilities all over the world, but after this there were more requests for help. I'm ready to help: I like to see the increasing body of evidence supporting our work. Not all studies are done well, but it is heartening to see so many people trying to investigate the field further. It was this, and a feeling not just from us but from others in the field that we need to encourage the highest standards of work, that led to us sponsoring and running a conference in 2015 of all the world leaders in the subject.

It seemed sense to get together: after all, it's silly to reinvent the wheel, and we can all profit from sharing our work and collaborating. Since our groundbreaking 2004 study, researchers across the world have woken up to the potential of dogs, and there is some very interesting bio-detection work going on. It was, predictably, John Church's idea, and the conference, which we named the Inaugural International Conference on Medical Bio Detection, was held at Emmanuel College, Cambridge, which is John's old college, in September 2015. Once again, we are indebted to Royal Canin for sponsoring the event, which attracted speakers from the Netherlands, the USA, Hawaii, Italy, Sweden, as well as from universities across Britain, including the Open University.

Rob Harris was there to give a demonstration with Ulric, Lucy and Midas, who was doing her first off-site demo. They all performed very well. After an introduction from John Church I gave the first talk. It was a lively day and a half, and a chance to exchange ideas with others working in the same field as us.

The conference made us all aware that we should work more collaboratively: after all, in this electronic age, distance is no barrier to sharing information. It was a unanimous decision that we should hold conferences again, probably every two years, and we set up a steering group to look at ways of sharing our work.

There is so much more to be done, and I am proud that we have ignited the interest that now spans the globe and which, I'm sure, will reap enormous rewards for mankind.

Tangle's death in October 2015 was a terrible time for me, but also a very moving event for everyone working at, and connected with, Medical Detection Dogs. We call him the dog who made history, because he was. He starred in the original studies that proved to a sceptical world that cancer has a smell, and that dogs can detect it. He was very focused, very calm, and nothing flustered him. He was always friendly with new people, but he constantly kept an eye on me, checking in. His silhouette, nose down, sniffing away, is enshrined forever on our literature and the red jackets our dogs wear. At the end of his life – he was thirteen and four months – he was an old man, grey round his muzzle, partially blind, very deaf, and no longer able to keep up with my other dogs. Eventually I faced the terrible decision that comes to all dog owners: is it fair to keep him alive? Am I selfishly allowing him to suffer so that I can still have his company?

It is never easy. When we take on dogs, we know that their lifespans are so much shorter than ours, and in a way we see in them a microcosm of our own mortality: the descent into frailty and old age. I mourned Tangle deeply, just as I have mourned all my dogs. But however much I loved him, and however extraordinary he was in terms of his ability and willingness to work, and his casual acceptance of all the publicity work he had to do, I never felt Tangle was quite one of my soul mates. There was something about him that remained slightly aloof, devoted to me but at the same time self-contained. Even at the end, when he was a lot more clingy to me, he didn't ask a lot from me, he was never demanding. He was always special, and I relied on him so much in the early days of our work, but it was almost as if it were on his terms. I remember how I felt when I went away, knowing that if anything happened to me, Tangle would accept being rehomed as long as he was well loved and looked after, whereas Woody and Daisy would pine away.

Looking back, Mr T came into my life when I still had Dill and Woody, and because Woody needed so much more from me, he accepted his place and trotted alongside, uncomplaining. There was something about him that was born mature: he never misbehaved, never wandered off; I never heard him bark. When he was really young I remember thinking that he wouldn't make old bones because he was already old beyond his years: thankfully I was wrong. When Rob, my boyfriend, joined our little pack he said to me: 'You don't treat Tangle like you treat Daisy and Woody, you don't talk to him the same.'

It wasn't conscious on my part: Tangle just didn't need me in the way the others did. Rob bonded with him, though, very strongly. Rob didn't have an easy childhood, and he was made to feel he was an outsider, so he empathised with Tangle, always saying when he arrived: 'Where's my little mate?'

As he got older and frailer, Tangle would stay with Rob while I went out for a run with the other dogs. Rob was distraught when he died, desperately upset. So it was to Rob that Tangle came back, in a dream, three or four days after his death. Rob sat bolt upright in bed, waking me up, and said: 'I've just seen Tangle. He was walking around, wagging his tail.'

Tangle had returned to say goodbye to his soul mate, and it wasn't me. I felt sad, but happy for Rob that he had another chance to say goodbye to his little mate, the dog who made history.

CHAPTER THIRTEEN

Postscript

'I can see the problem. His attention is all on finding food, and it's important to pair the food with what he has to do. He's motivated by the food, not by the search. He's got a split focus, and he has to know that finding the odour is his access to the food . . .'

Lydia was having trouble with a dog called Jack. She asked me to have a look at why he was slow to learn what we wanted him to do. He was being taught to find a tennis ball and a treat under pots that were laid out on the floor, in the way we worked at the very beginning of my experiments with dogs sniffing out cancer. Sometimes we still use the system with the diabetes-alert dogs. Eventually Jack will move on to a generalised diabetes odour. When he is good enough and reliable enough, he will progress to working with the specific odour of the person with diabetes he will eventually be paired with.

'He needs to know the odour means food, rather than searching for the odour of food,' I said to Lydia, who was using her clicker to tell Jack when he was getting it right.

However busy I am, I love these times when I am back to my roots, on the floor working with a dog, showing him what we need from him and watching for that wonderful moment when he picks up on it. As I've said before, all dogs are motivated slightly differently, so it is never a matter of training by rote, but of understanding the personality of the individual dog. We limit the amount of time each dog spends on training in a session, always stopping when they are doing well and getting rewards, rather than when they are failing and feeling deflated.

It's very important to me that I don't lose touch with training the dogs and being part of the front-line work, but at the same time I have to accommodate a slew of meetings about governance, finance and staffing, and I do publicity work and speaking engagements. It's a difficult balance.

The training staff are great, and I'm confident in delegating much of the work to them, but I'm never happier than when I am in the bio-detection room putting a dog through its paces. Daisy, my wonder dog, is always willing to work at her very high level for Rob and his team, although I fancy she gives that little bit extra when I am directing her. Eventually, of course, we will have more trainers working in bio detection, and we aim to have an even bigger team of dogs that will work equally for all of them.

I am always very involved in training when we are working on new projects to find different cancers. Then I am totally absorbed, puzzling out how to tell the dogs what odour we are looking for. It is still the part of our work that engages me the most; it's what wakes me in the night to run through new ideas in my head.

Medical Detection Dogs has a very simple message: we train dogs to detect human disease. Although there are now many more projects across the globe, we are still the world leaders, the pioneers. We are not following anyone, so every new development involves a great deal of time and thought, because there are no tried-and-tested systems to run with. I cannot visualise a day when I will say: my work is done.

When we had nothing, and not a spare penny in the bank, we got up in the morning and believed what we were doing would work. Day after day, with barely the money to pay anyone, and ranks of people dismissing us as cranks, all we had was our belief that we'd get somewhere, and what we were doing would one day be recognised as important. The people who were with me then are still with me, still believing, still giving everything to make this big idea of ours work.

Now that the organisation is bigger, expectations are higher, and the pressure is on. But we came from nothing, and our watchwords then are the same now: we want to be professional and compassionate at all times, and we have to keep focused on that. I want everyone who works here to be very proud of what we do. It's like ripples in a pond: you have to throw in a stone to get the ripple going, and then suddenly it has built into a huge wave, which gives the ability to do a lot more. But you have to start with the ripple, and then you must never let the wave swamp you.

When I look back, I can see that my relationship with animals is the thread that runs through my life, and finding a way to use our remarkable relationship with dogs is a journey I began years ago, and it is one that has a long way to go. We have learned so much, but the more we have learned the more we realise what huge potential is still untapped. There is hard work ahead, and exciting times as we make new discoveries.

I'm careful not to overstate what we do: there are other research projects round the world that claim they have cancer-detection dogs working at 98 per cent. I think it's possible to achieve this level with a brilliant dog like Daisy, but I don't believe it is possible to do it consistently with all dogs and a large sample size. I think it's important to be realistic, and I would never say that we can achieve more than a guaranteed success rate in the low nineties. Why boast of more? Ninety-three per cent is way ahead of most other screening tools, and we are doing it with a non-invasive, relatively cheap method. These dogs are not perfect, of course they aren't. But they are a whole lot better than anything else we have at present.

I welcome the fact that one day electronic noses may be developed to do the work we are doing with the dogs. But so far they are nowhere near the standards that we can achieve. Perhaps they never will get there. In the meantime, it would be so short-sighted not to harness the amazing gift our dogs give to medical science. Who know what more we will discover? Who knows what else they can show us, if we only take the time and trouble to understand the way they communicate with us?

One of my great hopes is that this work, as it spreads across the globe, will change attitudes to dogs in countries where they are treated with cruelty, disregard and lack of affection. When the abilities of dogs to help the human race are recognised, surely their status must improve? That, I believe, is one of the many powers of our work: it can change the lives of people with its huge health benefits, but also, I really hope, of dogs, too.

For me, personally, I have the most fulfilling career possible. My love of dogs has collided with my science brain, which is fascinated by them and what they can do. That's why I believe I was meant to do this job, and why everything that has happened to me has led me to where I am today.

Occasionally I think back to the teller in South Korea predicting that I would travel the world with my work. He was right: I have been to Canada, all over North America, Italy, Spain, Japan, Holland, Hawaii, Belgium, Germany, Norway, Portugal, Estonia, Poland . . . I'm sure there are more that I can't recall. I'm always happy to talk about my work and advise on other projects because I really believe the message about what dogs are capable of should be spread as far and as wide as possible.

I am very privileged to have shared my life with some exceptional dogs. At work and at home, I have their pictures on the walls around me, reminding me every day of the contribution these four-legged, waggy-tailed friends have made to medical science and the benefit of mankind. They have also brought love, companionship, laughter and fun into my life, seeing me through the darkest times and sharing my triumphs.

One of my great fears and sadnesses right now is that I know my beloved Daisy, who has worked and lived alongside me, who saved my life when she warned me of my cancer, is nearing the end of her natural lifespan. She is twelve years old, her muzzle is flecked with grey, her legs are a bit stiff when she gets up from her bed, and she's sleeping more than she did. However close we are to our dogs, however much we look after them, we cannot alter the fact that they will age in front of our eyes, and ultimately they will pass out of our lives. I have endured great misery when my dogs have died, and I dread it happening again, with Daisy.

There will be other dogs who will bring other things into my life, and I know I will never be without a four-legged furry companion. But there will never be another Daisy, just as there will never be another Ruffles, Dill, Woody or Tangle.

When Woody died, a friend sent me a card with a long printed message inside. I don't know who wrote the words, but I treasure them, and I read them over again whenever I lose one of my precious four-legged companions:

'Please do not cry for me. I am at rest now, no longer in pain. I have been restored to perfect health as I was intended to be . . . I sit in the lap of a familiar stranger, until we meet again, and our reunion will be great, filled with utter joy . . . Please do not think of me with sadness, think only of me with great love and adoration. I was sent to you as a gift, I came to you in a time and season when you needed me most. I, too, also needed you. I was sent to be your constant companion and confidante, this was my only task, and I asked nothing in return.

'It was my time to take leave of you . . . I am at peace now, and so shall you be. Deep within your heart, I live on, now and forever more. Please do not cry for me.'

I always do cry when I read it, for every dog that has ever shared my life and who, as the message says, lives on forever in my memories.

I owe everything to a very special line-up of dogs: Ruffles, Dill, Woody, Tangle and Daisy. I hope this book is a fitting tribute to them.

Acknowledgements

This book would not have happened without the support, encouragement and hard work of Piers Blofeld, Lorna Russell, Yvonne Jacob, Lucy Oates and Jean Ritchie. I also want to thank my family, who believed in me through the bad times and the good. Special thanks go to John Church, who inspired me and never lost faith. I can't underestimate the debt I owe to everyone who has supported the work of Medical Detection Dogs, through their work, through fundraising, through volunteering. Each and every one of you is part of this amazing story.